"*All I Eat Is Medicine* provides a powerful critique of global public health in the key context of HIV/AIDS treatment scale-up in Africa. Ippolytos Kalofonos brilliantly traces legacies of colonialism, war, racism, extraction, and international development as they affect personal and collective experiences of hunger and sickness. He presents flesh-and-blood accounts of people in Mozambique living with HIV/AIDS as they navigate the emerging AIDS economy and care for one another as community health workers, volunteers, and activists. Witnessing the inspiring actions of individuals, families, and communities, Kalofonos contributes one of the most compelling critiques of the 'biomedical tunnel vision' that effaces political, economic, and social realities in a stifling focus on individual behavior. Building on the work of social medicine visionary Frantz Fanon, Kalofonos calls for global solidarity in moving beyond the provision of medicine and confronting the political and economic forces, institutions, and policies that produce social and health inequities in the first place. *All I Eat Is Medicine* is a must-read for everyone who cares about health, medicine, social inequities, and global relations."

Seth M. Holmes, University of California, Berkeley, author of *Fresh Fruit, Broken Bodies*

"Through careful observations and intimate narratives drawn from long-term fieldwork, this valuable ethnography shows that the scaling up of HIV treatment in Mozambique altered ordinary lives in unintended ways. Kalofonos reveals how a successful global-health intervention can also be a betrayal, and a medication side effect can be a potent political critique."

Claire Wendland, University of Wisconsin-Madison, author of *A Heart for the Work*

"Weaving together compelling case studies and a persuasive argument, *All I Eat Is Medicine* offers sensitive ethnographic portrayals and illuminating analysis. Written in clear and accessible prose, the book speaks to both a medical anthropology audience and a wider public."

Daniel Jordan Smith, Professor of Anthropology, Brown University

"*All I Eat Is Medicine* examines the rise of global health at a unique moment and from a rare vantage point. Its chronicle of the lives and struggles of people living with HIV and AIDS in Mozambique demonstrates how long-term fieldwork can marshal powerful insights into the life-and-death stakes that emerged as the first generation of ARV treatment programs were rolled out in Africa. It serves as a model for medical anthropology and offers an accessible and moving account of interest to students and practitioners of global health."

Vinh-Kim Nguyen, Co-Director, Global Health Centre,
The Graduate Institute, Geneva

"Searingly honest, *All I Eat* offers an eye-opening, deeply grounded analysis of the perils of global-health reductionism. Foregrounding the jarring voices of activists and other people living with HIV/AIDS, Kalofonos argues that unless embedded power asymmetries are shattered and replaced by a truly collaborative 'ethics of interdependence,' the intertwining problems of disease, hunger, and poverty will persist, wonder drugs notwithstanding."

Anne-Emanuelle Birn, University of Toronto, lead author of Oxford's
Textbook of Global Health

"Physician-anthropologist Ippy Kalofonos masterfully reworks metaphors of African hunger and international medical relief to show how colonization is alive and well in global pharmaceutical regimes. A must-read for anyone who wants to understand the biomedical basis of contemporary racial capitalism—and, more importantly, for anyone who wants to stop it."

Helena Hansen, MD PhD, Professor, David Geffen School of Medicine,
University of California, Los Angeles

"In *All I Eat Is Medicine*, Ippolytos Kalofonos makes a clarion call for a Global Health agenda that goes beyond the technological 'magic bullets' of antiretroviral drug distribution to one based on the values of ethnographic intimacy, care, social solidarity, inclusion, equity, and social and medical justice."

Nancy Scheper-Hughes, author of *Death without Weeping: The
Violence of Everyday Life in Brazil*

All I Eat Is Medicine

All I Eat Is Medicine

GOING HUNGRY IN MOZAMBIQUE'S
AIDS ECONOMY

Ippolytos Kalofonos

UNIVERSITY OF CALIFORNIA PRESS

University of California Press
Oakland, California

© 2021 by Ippolytos Kalofonos

Library of Congress Cataloging-in-Publication Data

Names: Kalofonos, Ippolytos, author.
Title: All I eat is medicine : going hungry in Mozambique's AIDS
    economy / Ippolytos Kalofonos.
Other titles: California series in public anthropology ; 52.
Description: Oakland, California : University of California Press, [2021] |
    Series: California series in public anthropology ; 52 | Includes
    bibliographical references and index.
Identifiers: LCCN 2021006467 (print) | LCCN 2021006468 (ebook) |
    ISBN 9780520289390 (cloth) | ISBN 9780520289406 (paperback) |
    ISBN 9780520964075 (epub)
Subjects: LCSH: AIDS (Disease)—Social aspects—Mozambique—
    21st century. | AIDS (Disease)—Economic aspects—Mozambique—
    21st century. | AIDS (Disease)—Patients—Mozambique—21st century.
Classification: LCC RA643.86.M85 K35 2021 (print) |
    LCC RA643.86.M85 (ebook) | DDC 362.19697/92009679—dc23
LC record available at https://lccn.loc.gov/2021006467
LC ebook record available at https://lccn.loc.gov/2021006468

Manufactured in the United States of America

30 29 28 27 26 25 24 23 22 21
10 9 8 7 6 5 4 3 2 1

For my parents, Vanna-Maria and Dionysios

Contents

Figures

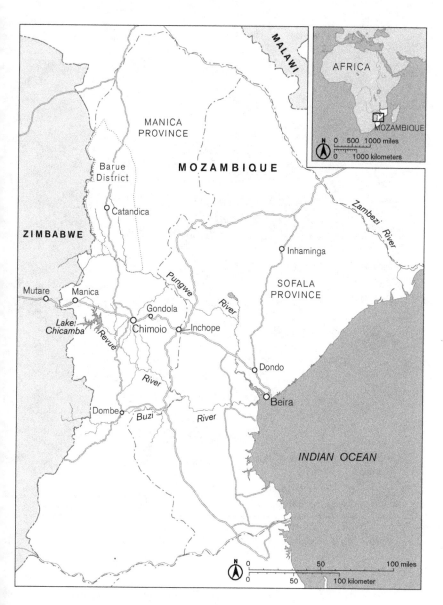

Map 1. Central Mozambique. Drawn by Ben Pease.

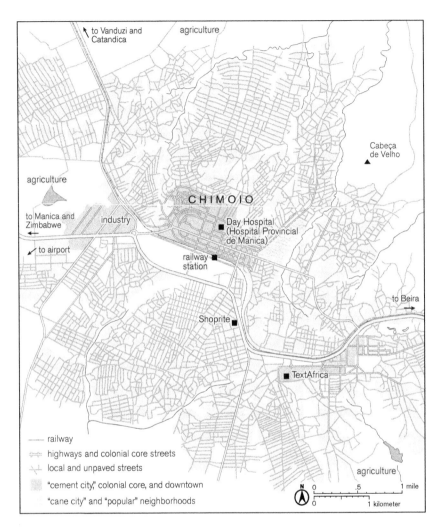

Map 2. Chimoio. Drawn by Ben Pease.

Introduction

A DOENÇA DO SÉCULO
(THE DISEASE OF THE CENTURY)

This book examines a key period in the global AIDS pandemic, between 2003 and 2010, when treatment for AIDS was finally made available on a broad scale in southern Africa. This was an important event for Mozambique, where HIV was estimated to have infected a staggering 16.2 percent of the overall population and as high as 25 percent in the country's hotspots.[1] Treatment for HIV/AIDS was developed and made available in the global north in the mid-1990s, but it was beyond the reach of much of the global south due to cost and "technical requirements." In the absence of treatment, HIV was taking a catastrophic toll on Mozambique. The scale-up of treatment in Mozambique should therefore have been a time of celebration and rejuvenation. But the story was—and is—not so simple.

Indeed, scholars, the media, and health and development organizations did and do celebrate this scale-up of HIV testing, care, and treatment in Africa. The scale-up is seen as a remarkable story of contemporary humanitarian intervention and the signature triumph

1

of "the new global health."[2] The World Health Organization (WHO) sponsored a campaign it called "3 x 5" that expressed the goals of the intervention numerically: to treat no fewer than three million individuals by 2005. In Mozambique, one of the poorest countries in the world as well as one of the ten countries most heavily impacted by the pandemic, the number of people on treatment increased from a mere 3,000 in 2003 to over 300,000 a decade later.[3]

The undeniable benefits of AIDS treatment were publicized in dramatic before-and-after pictures demonstrating what is called the *Lazarus effect*: a gaunt, hollow-eyed body at death's door is transformed by antiretroviral medication, or "ARVs," into a full-fleshed, smiling, healthy individual with a future, a renewal akin to Jesus's resurrection of his dead friend Lazarus in the New Testament.[4] Fundraising and public health campaigns used these images internationally to raise money and support for the rollout of medication.[5] The dramatic imagery of the Lazarus effect and the rising count of lives saved portrayed an unmitigated success story of high-tech treatment provided in an impoverished setting and fueled talk of "the end of AIDS."[6]

Beyond the bare fact of survival, the numbers and images tell us little about how life changed for people living in the areas impacted by AIDS and targeted by the treatment interventions. Missing in the narrative of biological recovery are the relationships—between individuals, social groups, organizations, and sovereign powers—that shape the longer trajectory of global AIDS treatment interventions as well as the meaning and value of survival. This book, then, goes beyond the imagery and numbers of "lives saved" to provide flesh-and-blood accounts of people living with AIDS at the start of the treatment era. It embeds these accounts within the broader story of social change that shapes the emergent framework of diagnosis, treatment, health, and disease.[7] This book places AIDS treatment within local moral and political economies of care and argues that by disregarding the material realities of collective survival and providing a medical treatment focused solely on biological life, this massive global health intervention established new forms of suffering and subjection. Even as it saved lives, the AIDS treatment scale-up perpetuated the exploitation and exclusion that was implicated in the propagation of the epidemic in the first place. This book calls attention to the global social commitments and responsibilities that a truly therapeutic global health requires.

PANDEMIC HOTSPOT: AIDS IN CENTRAL MOZAMBIQUE

Central Mozambique is a regional crossroads that emerged as a hotspot for the AIDS pandemic. While the first AIDS case in Mozambique was reported in 1986, there was little population data available throughout the 1980s. A civil war ravaged the country from 1977 to 1992, consuming the majority of available resources and destroying much of the health and transportation infrastructure required for such surveillance. With the signing of the cease-fire in 1992 and the return of many of the displaced (*deslocados*), often from refugee camps in high-prevalence settings of neighboring countries, what statistics were available indicated that HIV prevalence quickly increased.[8] In 1994, Chimoio—capital city of the province of Manica—had one of the highest rates of HIV in the country at 10.7 percent, likely due to the city's position on one of southeastern Africa's main transport routes, the Beira corridor, which links Zimbabwe in the west to the eastern port city of Beira. It is estimated that between 1993 and 1996, nearly half of the Mozambican population was in transit along such routes, including the *deslocados* and 270,000 demobilized soldiers.[9] The Beira corridor was also traversed by Zimbabwean and then UN peacekeeping troops in the aftermath of the war. These population movements accelerated HIV transmission, and the central region became home to 52.2 percent of all Mozambicans living with HIV/AIDS, despite comprising just 42 percent of the national population.[10] Infection rates were exceptionally high in towns and cities, with rates estimated to be at around a quarter of the adult population in Chimoio at the time of my fieldwork.[11] These infection rates made Mozambique one of the nine African countries hardest hit by the HIV/AIDS epidemic and the central region one of the epicenters of the global AIDS pandemic. AIDS was popularly known as "the disease of the century," or "*a doença do século*," because of the scale of the impact and the timing of the epidemic's arrival in the public consciousness at the turn of the millennium.

THE ARRIVAL OF AIDS TREATMENT

I arrived in Mozambique in 2003, when HIV testing was expanding nationally and planning was underway for the scale-up of antiretroviral therapy. As a student of both medicine and anthropology, I was drawn to Mozambique to learn how global health interventions were taken up on a local level. I had spent much of my undergraduate and medical school education learning about the unjust global distribution of ARVs. When I learned in the spring of 2003 that AIDS testing in Mozambique was just being scaled up and treatment was on the horizon, I was excited by the opportunity to be on the ground.

The AIDS treatment scale-up was a watershed moment for public health in Mozambique, and indeed globally. Free AIDS treatment, in the form of ARVs, was finally a reality for the Mozambican National Health Service (NHS). Even though ARVs had been developed in 1995, effectively transforming a fatal illness into a chronic disease in North America and Europe, the cost of these medications kept them out of the hands of most people living in low-income countries, including the majority of those who lived in southeastern Africa. In the early 2000s, however, thanks in part to global activism and advocacy, unprecedented amounts of funding flowed from organizations such as the World Bank; the Global Fund to Fight AIDS,

Tuberculosis, and Malaria; the Clinton Foundation; and the President's Emergency Plan for AIDS Relief (PEPFAR).[12] Funding for HIV/AIDS in Mozambique increased thirtyfold from 2003 to 2007, going from around US$3 million in 2002 to around $50 million in 2004, $70 million in 2005, and $110 million in 2006.[13] PEPFAR's budget would ultimately match the entire budget of Mozambique's ministry of health.[14] PEPFAR's goal over its first five years of existence (2004–2008) was similar to the goal of the WHO campaign, to meet narrowly defined numerical targets legislated by the US Congress: treat two million people with antiretroviral treatment, prevent seven million new infections, and offer care to ten million people infected with or affected by HIV/AIDS.[15] This largesse would be channeled to predominantly US-based nongovernmental organizations (NGOs) rather than to public sector health systems, in accordance with the constraints imposed to support privatization as part of the broader neoliberal shift in Africa.[16] Thus, this investment did not result in expanded health systems in the recipient countries.[17]

While the imperative to treat HIV/AIDS in southeastern Africa was clear, the ways institutions, technologies, and vast resources were mobilized in the implementation of treatment programs proved to have mixed results. I was particularly interested in how access to limited resources would be negotiated and how the biomedical categories and technologies associated with the AIDS treatment interventions would alter people's self-conceptions and relationships with others.[18] An impressive interdisciplinary scholarship has documented the ways inequality drives the spread of HIV.[19] Inequality also influences the ways that states and global actors do and do not respond to the AIDS pandemic.[20] Studies of early AIDS treatment interventions emphasized how technologies were deployed globally according to logics of governance and population management.[21] This book details how the treatment interventions themselves reinforced existing inequalities when the influx of resources specifically for AIDS treatment contributed to the emergence of an AIDS economy.

The AIDS economy emerged at the intersections of a local therapeutic economy, the threadbare national health system, and the
neoliberal development economy that had been imposed on Mozambique in the wake of the civil war.[22] This economic shift from socialism was required by the International Monetary Fund (IMF) and
the World Bank in order for Mozambique, which had been bank-
rupted by the war, to receive economic aid. It involved the largest
privatization program in sub-Saharan Africa in the 1990s and had
a profound effect on the way AIDS treatment was delivered.[23] The
private sector—rather than government—was called on to provide
health services. In this environment, international donors funded
AIDS treatment interventions through NGOs, who partnered with
government health services to provide free medical treatment, food
aid, employment, support for orphans and vulnerable children, and
access to additional initiatives related to AIDS education and care
to those who had a documented HIV positive diagnosis. AIDS treatment interventions created a dynamic sphere of exchange related to
AIDS, within which individuals maneuvered and negotiated. This
AIDS economy reinforced existing inequalities and created new
hierarchies, even as lives were saved.[24]

THE LAZARUS EFFECT AND
THE SOCIAL BASIS OF HEALING

The image of the Lazarus effect communicates a miraculous simplic-
ity: a pill, delivered from far away, dramatically restores vitality. This
simple, individualized narrative of a person and a pill obscures the
social basis of health, healing, and personhood in central Mozambique—and indeed elsewhere.[25] Across Africa, concepts of sociality
and circulation underlie the notions of proper living; "the person"
is not conceptualized as an independent entity but rather is constituted through pro-social relationships.[26] In contrast to neoliberal
ideals of independence and self-reliance, personhood is understood

to be achieved through relationships with others.[27] These relations are often governed by what anthropologist China Scherz, working in Uganda, has termed an "ethics of interdependence."[28] This means that "people with resources stand to gain from their relationships with people who have less; that they have a moral obligation to take on clients; and that people with limited resources must actively try to attach themselves to more powerful others as dependents."[29] This interdependence is based on mutually reciprocal sets of obligations and responsibilities. Anthropologists have termed the logic of such systems, in which political leaders become powerful by amassing followers, "wealth in people."[30] A client might provide labor or political support, while a patron might provide livelihood and protection. As patrons compete for clients, clients are free to move between patrons in order to meet their needs, leading to anthropologist James Ferguson's observation that the "freedom that existed in such a social world . . . came not from independence, but from a plurality of opportunities for dependence."[31]

These notions of personhood and the ethics and morality of social life undergird basic assumptions about health and healing. Historian-anthropologist Steven Feierman masterfully lays out this thesis in his extensive review of the social context of health and healing in modern Africa.[32] Similarly, anthropologist Jean Comaroff characterized all forms of healing as cultural products that represent "human intervention in disorder—culturally specific self-conscious attempts to mend the physical, emotional, and social breaches caused by illness."[33] Physician-anthropologist Michael Taussig has argued, for example, that biomedical doctors working under capitalist conditions in the United States view disease as a biomedical object separate from social relations, rendering illness an individual, private experience and masking the social conditions, be they poverty or prejudice, out of which illness emerges and which shape its trajectory.[34] While the onset of illness often brings to light contradictions in the social order, healing processes reinforce meanings and interpretations that reflect the vision of reality of specific social interests.

While biomedicine targets pathology in the individual body and brackets it out as a biological event, healing in sub-Saharan Africa has historically been "public, collective, and imbued with moral purpose."[35] Illness in Mozambique can have several etiologies, which influence how and where it might be made visible and where care might be sought. In popular narratives and among traditional healers in central Mozambique, illnesses are regarded as "natural" or "provoked."[36] Malaria and cholera, for example, are considered "natural." Most diseases, however, are provoked, or "sent." These diseases have a relational origin because they result from the active, purposeful intervention of an agent, who might be human or supernatural.[37] Relational illnesses are attributed to witchcraft or sorcery (*uroi*), an evil spirit (*espírito mau*), or ancestral spirits (*vadzimu*). *Uroi* might come from a woman who hosts the spirit of a maternal ancestor endowed with special powers that can either heal or harm, or from someone, more frequently a man, who purchases powerful medicine (*mutombo*) to harm someone or amass personal benefit and wealth at the expense of others. Alternatively, those who fail to follow proper social norms and behavior might succumb to diseases because *vadzimu* withdraw their protection from someone who has been immoral, either through infidelity or the creation of family conflict, or from someone who has failed to follow ritual patterns of respect toward elders.[38] In addition, avenging spirits (*mupfukwa*), especially the spirits of the victims of murder or past wars, might provoke illnesses to settle scores that could be generations old.[39] These spirits can be harnessed and directed to harm rivals and enemies.[40] Therapeutic power is therefore considered highly ambivalent, with the power to harm as well as heal.

Treating illnesses provoked by spiritual affliction is the domain of herbalist healer-diviners (*n'angas*), who may have multiple spirits at their disposal, or prophet-healers (*profetes*), whose healing powers come from the Holy Spirit and are integrated within a Christian framework. A *n'anga* can be possessed by and at the mercy of these spirits.[41] The *n'anga* elicits the power of a spirit in a ritual setting to diagnose the cause of an affliction and attempt to treat it, at the individual or collective level. A *profete* typically holds a prominent position within a local church.

N'angas and *profetes* make their diagnoses by looking not only at the sick body of an individual, but also at that individual's relationships with kin, alive and dead, and the natural world.[42] Health and illness are seen as broad concepts for harmony and disruption, and healing is often oriented toward mending social rupture. Such a conception of health implies a set of interdependencies, obligations, and expectations between kin, between the more and less powerful, between leaders and subjects, between patrons and clients, and between the social and the natural worlds.

"ALL I EAT IS ARVS": HUNGER AND AIDS TREATMENT

AIDS was often initially diagnosed as a provoked illness, but eventually relatively well-funded treatment programs enticed the ill to seek medical intervention alongside traditional sources of healing. People recovering from AIDS looked to these sites of global intervention not only for the medication that prolonged their lives but also for sources of income to bolster their devastated livelihoods. While access to medication expanded, the material support for living—employment or food, for example—proved more elusive. While people on ARVs regained their health, and in some cases became healthy for the first time in months or years, they also regained their appetites. This hunger was an index of bodies returning to health but also threw a stark light onto the fact that there was very little support available for survival beyond medication. The Lazarus effect—recovering from AIDS, thanks to advanced medical care—betrayed the reality of the bodily and social experience of living with HIV/AIDS. The reality was that individuals on ARVs were tormented by an unrelenting hunger. The irony of surviving AIDS just to suffer from hunger was not lost on survivors, and they talked about this frequently.

During a break from a seminar about ARV treatment in an association of people living with HIV/AIDS, a handful of attendees were recounting some of the dramatic recoveries they had experienced and witnessed. Florência, who had nearly been given up for dead before accessing treatment, was celebrating her recovery with the association she belonged to.[43] Another woman had commented: "There's Florência, she is strong, strong! She really got fat. Florência! God has helped you! God has helped you my friend, you really are well! I'm not lying, look at you!" In this context, "fat" did not mean rotund, chubby, or large-bellied. It meant healthy and no longer emaciated. And yet, as peals of laughter punctuated the conversation and we shared thin slices of spiny cucumbers and salt, stomachs grumbled:

FLORÊNCIA: I wake up at midnight to eat!

MANUEL: "Do you know what it is for your organism [your body] to be asking for food? It wakes me in the middle of the night, and I have to eat!"

FLORÊNCIA: "This treatment really causes hunger!"

MANUEL: "Don't you know why? The body needs food in order to recover. The organism demands it!"

FLORÊNCIA: "What can I do? I have nothing to eat. All I eat is ARVs!"

Florência and Manuel continued to talk about the hunger that accompanied their recovery. The hunger woke them up in the middle of the night. Manuel spoke of "the organism" and "the body" demanding food, like a force out of control, a voracious beast, or a greedy master. In households that constantly struggled to feed all their members, this hunger was not only painful but socially disruptive and unwelcome. Manuel referred to his body as if it were separate from him, as if to say it was not he himself asking for more food, but his "organism" and his pills. What does it mean to provide a treatment that bundles hunger with its biological therapy? Do we consider the medication to be therapeutically efficacious—or do we insist that the therapy solve the problem it uncovers or creates? What kind of life can be led under these conditions? What does it mean to provide medical treatment that inflicts hunger in a setting of widespread malnutrition?

Amid short-term project goals and contracts, tallies of numbers treated and lives saved, the AIDS treatment programs appeared to be quite blind to the realities of living with ARVs. This hunger exposed the way AIDS treatment interventions had effects that were not only biological but profoundly political as well. In Mozambique, as in much of Africa, idioms of hunger and eating are used as an embodied moral language to address issues of sociality, justice, inequality, privilege, and power. Historian Jean-François Bayart coined the phrase "the politics of the belly" to refer to processes of and drives for material accumulation as well as the symbolic association of eating with political domination.[44] Anthropologist Harry West notes that his informants in northern Mozambique "have long expressed ambivalence toward power in the idiom of consumption . . . [T]hey acrimoniously described the powerful in their midst . . . as 'those who eat well' or 'those who eat everything.'"[45] Interpreted within an ethics of interdependence, the powerful who eat well also have an obligation to feed others. Power that provides collective wealth and prosocial prosperity is spoken of as "feeding the people."[46] Antisocial, exploitative wealth, gained illegitimately at the expense of others and not redistributed, is referred to as "eating the food of others" and discussed using metaphors of cannibalism, bloodsucking, and witchcraft.[47] Witches are said to eat alone and to eat human flesh, accumulating vitality for their own personal benefit, the ultimate act of destructive, antisocial selfishness.

Florência's exasperated exclamation at the association meeting— "All I eat is ARVs"—can be interpreted within this context. Talk of hunger is a commentary on both individual, physiological sensations and social and political dynamics of distribution and exchange that are at the heart of health, well-being, and survival. Florência understood herself to be in a relationship with those who provided treatment that entailed reciprocal obligations. She was adhering to her treatment regimen and struggled to enact the changes in her life that AIDS treatment programs demanded. In exchange she expected to be cared for. How could it be that she was left hungry? Her hunger was indicative of the failure of AIDS treatment interventions to adequately provide care.

The coexistence of hunger and HIV in Mozambique did not necessarily come as a surprise. What was surprising was this claim that ARVs *caused* or at the very least worsened that hunger, and in the context of the triumphal spirit of the scale-up, statements from patients that all they had to eat was pills was chilling. People living with HIV who were already hungry feared initiating and often abandoned treatment. Because ARVs incited hunger, and treatment programs did not provide enough food to assuage it, the programs were seen as antisocial—generating suspicion, competition, and illness. The vast majority of people I encountered who were on ARV treatment were grateful for the life it granted them, but through the language of hunger they also expressed profound ambivalence regarding the treatment programs. On the one hand, hunger signified a restless affirmation of life, of the healthy body restored. It could be mobilized as a motivating force toward action. Indeed, initiating and staying on treatment would require immense individual and collective labor, as the following chapters document. Nevertheless, this came with a profound disappointment with how the treatment programs inflicted but did not resolve this persistent hunger.

If, as the philosopher Juan Manuel Garrido maintains, "politics is nothing other than the promise of alleviating hunger," we might understand these complaints of persistent hunger as indicative of political failure.[48] While the Mozambican invocation of hunger as an idiom socialized and politicized the bodily sensation, the treatment programs individualized it and medicalized it. In this way, AIDS treatment could be seen as functioning as an "antipolitics machine": hunger was reduced to a technical problem that might interfere with the narrow goal of AIDS treatment rather than a social and political problem implicated in the constitution of the epidemic itself.[49]

THE BIOPOLITICS OF THE AIDS TREATMENT SCALE-UP

While the language of the "scale-up"—terminology used by organizations implementing the AIDS treatment programs, such as the WHO and the Joint United Nations HIV/AIDS Program (UNAIDS)—was predominantly technocratic and guided by quantitative measures, important social and political effects resulted from the ways AIDS treatment was implemented in Mozambique.[50] Inasmuch as AIDS treatment interventions aimed to change behavior, they enacted a form of politics directed toward the shaping of a particular kind of person and society. This perspective is informed by Michel Foucault's analysis of modern European state power. He introduced the term *biopower* to designate forms of power exercised over persons as living beings, a politics concerned with subjects as members of a population, connecting matters of biology, sexuality, and reproduction to national policy and power.[51] The exercise of biopower, which Foucault termed *governmentality*, deploys a range of technologies that target, describe, and seek to regulate specific populations, giving rise to forms of life that were previously unknown.[52] Race is integral to biopower, as a means of separating and categorizing a population, establishing a naturalized hierarchy of value, and then identifying groups to "make live" and to "let die" for the health of the overall population.[53] Race was a central trope of colonialism and persists in contemporary development and global health regimes, albeit in submerged form.[54]

Biomedical interventions can powerfully shape people's subjectivities, the ways they think about themselves and relate to others.[55] Emphasizing this latter dynamic, anthropologist Paul Rabinow termed the process in which a shared biological condition may foster new forms of belonging *biosociality*.[56] Building on these concepts, anthropologists have charted the emergence of forms of political belonging in which access to social welfare benefits, previously conferred on all citizens of the state, is predicated on biological status or a medical diagnosis.[57] These claims of biologically based rights are made on transnational actors like NGOs, international governmental bodies, and pharmaceutical companies. In her ethnography of the aftermath of the Chernobyl nuclear disaster, anthropologist Adriana Petryna defines biological citizenship as "a massive demand for but selective access to a form of social welfare based on medical, scientific, and legal criteria that both acknowledge biological injury and compensate for it."[58] Working in West Africa, Vinh-Kim Nguyen describes a form of therapeutic citizenship in which the HIV diagnosis provides individuals with "access to forms of material security one usually associates with citizenship."[59] In both of these cases, "thin" forms of citizenship are provided by transnational institutions when the existing state is unable or unwilling to provide resources like health care.[60] In light of these observations, my aim was to document and analyze how the new technologies, practices, and discourses related to AIDS treatment would be taken up in central Mozambique. How would these treatment interventions shape the subjectivities of those receiving treatment?[61] What kinds of relationships, or biosocialities, would emerge among the subjects of these interventions, who were brought together by their common biological predicament? What does the outcome of persistent hunger mean for the politics of global health?

LIVING POSITIVELY IN THE AIDS ECONOMY

AIDS treatment interventions brought together a complex assemblage of drug delivery systems, biomedical technologies, institutions, and authorities. Health and illness were individual, biological traits, measured and assessed through clinical exams and blood tests, and the priority was treating AIDS and preventing HIV from spreading. The interventions operated according to the logics of not just biomedicine and individualism but also the neoliberal values of entrepreneurialism, competition, privatization, and decentralization. AIDS treatment programs valorized and rewarded those who could embody the virtues of self-actualization, personal autonomy, responsibility, enterprise, choice, and future-orientation. They contributed to the shaping of a particular kind of subject, one able to follow the advice of counselors and clinicians; adhere to antiretroviral medications; practice self-care, monogamy, and condom use; plan for the future; assume responsibility for one's own health and future; and speak out about their status as HIV positive—precepts that together were known as "positive living," or "living positively" (*Vida Positiva*). Those who could or would not meet these criteria were seen as not deserving treatment. The AIDS treatment interventions brought into being the sphere of therapy, care, and exchange that I refer to as the AIDS economy.

I use the term *AIDS economy* throughout this book to describe the way the medicalization and individualization of health, mediated by health systems, NGOs, and external donors through AIDS treatment interventions, interacted with broader social and political notions of health, healing, and well-being in the context of an ongoing subsistence crisis in central Mozambique.[62] The concept of the AIDS economy evokes social historian E. P. Thompson's concept of a "moral economy," which he developed while analyzing the food riots that broke out in eighteenth-century England in response to the emerging capitalist market's violation of customary norms and practices.[63] A *moral economy* is a system of norms and obligations, defined by a local world of values, that informs expectations about appropriate behavior and guides judgments and actions.[64] The notion of the moral economy was developed to highlight the opposition between the universal "maximizing individual and ever-expanding market of classical political economy" on the one hand, and an economy deeply embedded in local social activity, governed by norms of collective survival, and existing in a zero-sum universe, a world where all profit is gained at someone else's expense.[65] Thompson's concern with unequal class relations and his focus on the role of the marketplace as a site of class conflict and struggle is also relevant for Mozambique, as the treatment scale-up proceeded in a context of increasing inequality resulting from neoliberal reform.[66] I use the term AIDS economy in order to point to the disjuncture between the expectations engendered by the medicalized and individualized conception of health underlying the logic of the AIDS treatment interventions, on the one hand, and the expectations held by the recipients and users, who historically have held a broader social and relational view of health, and whose moral economies of care differ substantially from the assumptions of the AIDS economy.

The arrival of AIDS treatment interventions, administered though government health clinics and NGOs and supported by an array of outreach, education, and care initiatives, changed the economic and moral value of HIV in ways that resonated with the ideologies of regnant neoliberalism as well as those of local Pentecostal churches, which proliferated in Mozambique during this period of neoliberal economic reform. Many people living with HIV/AIDS in Mozambique saw themselves as members and evangelists of a new "church," of *Vida Positiva*, living positively with AIDS. In order to materially benefit in the AIDS economy—that is, to receive free antiretroviral medication as well as the possibility of food support, employment, and access to a network of AIDS-related support interventions and organizations—individuals had to demonstrate that they adhered to certain values and behaviors. This resulted in competition, resentment, and increased social division.[67] By focusing on saving individual lives as the desired outcome of the intervention, the underlying factors of poverty and hunger were unaddressed and, in some ways, exacerbated. AIDS treatment interventions themselves created an economy that reinforced contemporary realities of increasing scarcity, inequality, competition, and uncertainty for both people living with AIDS and those who stepped forward to care for them.

THE CITY OF CHIMOIO

I conducted the majority of my participant-observation fieldwork in and around Chimoio, the fifth largest city in Mozambique and capital of the central province of Manica. A regional hotspot of the AIDS pandemic, the city was a hub of many early HIV/AIDS interventions, including community home-based care volunteer networks, associations of people living with HIV/AIDS, AIDS specialty clinics called "Day Hospitals," and pilot programs for testing and treatment. Though the dominant local language is Chitewe, immigrants from all over Mozambique and Zimbabwe have made Chimoio a multiethnic, multilingual city. The majority speak both Chitewe and the former colonial language Portuguese.[68]

Mount Bengo, a large rock whose summit rises two hundred meters high, is one of Chimoio's most prominent features. Viewed from the east and west, it looks like the profile of an old man; its Portuguese name is, in fact, Old Man's Head (Cabeça do Velho). Ancestral spirits inhabit the mountain, and it is a site of ritual importance.[69] Visible from Bengo's summit are the tall buildings of Chimoio's city center, the former colonial center known as the cement city (*cidade de cimento*), and the sprawling cane city (*cidade de caniço*), named for the characteristic thatched roofs of most of the dwellings, where the majority of residents live. Entering the city from national highway EN6 (Estrada Nacional 6), travelers pass

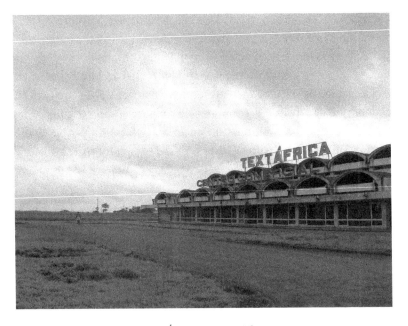

Figure 1. The now defunct TextÁfrica commercial center.

the shuttered industrial complex TextÁfrica, the textile mill once at the heart of a vibrant company town (see figure 1). A new strip mall is just two kilometers further down the highway. In contrast to TextÁfrica, it is brightly lit and bustling, anchored by Shoprite Chimoio, a South African supermarket chain, which is flanked by retail shops, fast-food franchises, a travel agency, and a parking lot that is surrounded by a high fence and patrolled by security guards. The Worker's Plaza (Praça dos Trabalhadores) stands at the intersection where the EN6 meets another road entering the city. The Praça dos Trabalhadores is marked by a concrete slab depicting two stick figures clasping each other's shoulders, each raising a hoe toward a red star above them, a monument from Mozambique's socialist period. Emblematic of the changing times, a recent addition had been made in red paint on the base of the monument: "Mozambican Workers

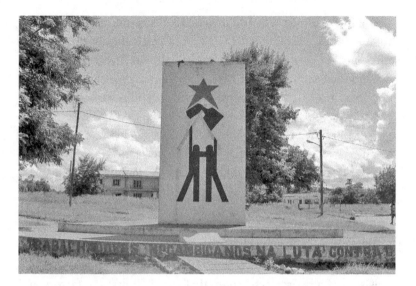

Figure 2. Monument in the Praça dos Trabalhadores, Chimoio.

Engaged in the Fight Against HIV/AIDS" (*Trabalhadores Moçambicanos Na Luta Contra O HIV/SIDA*) (see figure 2).

Renamed Chimoio at independence, the colonial city of Vila Pery was constructed around the railway station built in 1893. The city was well positioned along the railway between Beira and Zimbabwe and between the Pungwe and Revue Rivers to become the center of a regional colonial economy based on agriculture. Settlers, attracted to the region by the railway and favorable climate, appropriated the most fertile lands. These settlers came not only from Portugal but also from Greece, Italy, France, Germany, Great Britain, South Africa, India, and China.[70] By 1911, there were fifty-one settler farms around Chimoio and forty-six farther west, around Vila Manica.[71] Tax laws forced African farmers off their lands by requiring payment in European currency or labor, creating a pool of cheap workers compelled to work on European plantations or in the nascent light industrial sector.

Following World War II, Portugal launched an industrialization initiative as an attempt to justify its continued colonization. The Cotton Society of Portugal (Sociedade Algodeira de Portugal, SOALPO), was founded in Portugal in 1944. Chimoio was chosen as a factory site because of its location in the Beira corridor, the proximity of the railway and rivers, and the burgeoning European settlement, with at the time around a thousand Europeans living in Chimoio.[72] An industrial complex covering a little over eight and a half acres was built, including the complete elements for the entire production cycle of cotton, as well as a residential park extension, a village annex for *indígena* (indigenous, native African) workers, primary schools for whites and *indígena*, a chapel, a hospital, and a sports and recreation club. The Hydroelectric Society of the Revuè (Sociedade Hidro-Eléctrica do Revuè, SHER) was also established, which consisted of a hydroelectric dam that supplied first the factory and later the entire region with electrical power. SOALPO was renamed TextÁfrica at independence and operated throughout the postwar period, with occasional interruptions, before closing in 2002.

The *cidade de cimento* (see figure 3) consisted of a grid of paved streets with concrete buildings housing government offices, banks, a commercial center with restaurants and shops, upper-middle-class apartments and homes, hotels, schools, the provincial hospital, the railway station, several informal markets, an imposing neo-Gothic Catholic cathedral, and an enormous green-and-white mosque with four minarets. Where the pavement and orderly grid of the *cidade de cimento* ended, the *cidade de caniço* began, with its crisscrossing dirt roads. These roads were often nothing more than dusty footpaths (*picadas*) that become muddy bogs in the rain. While garbage accumulated in the gullies and gutters—desiccated corn cobs and sugar cane, plastic debris, empty blister packs and pill bottles—front yards, or *quintals*, were swept clean as residents sought to impose what order they could. The poorer neighborhoods (*bairros*; also called *bairros populares*, popular neighborhoods) usually lacked electricity and running water. The vast majority of Chimoio's inhabitants lived

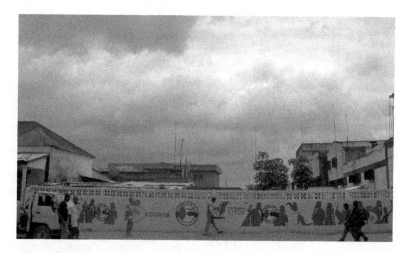

Figure 3. Busy street in the *cidade de cimento.*

in these *bairros*, in houses of mud brick with the *cidade de caniço* roofs of thatched vegetation or, less often, of corrugated zinc (see figure 4). Many of these *bairros* were formed during the civil war as rural residents sought the relative safety of the city, though a couple of relatively affluent *bairros* had been more recently constructed. The *bairros populares* were crowded and bustling with blaring radios and the buzz of conversation, laughter, shouts, and arguments. Chimoio's neighborhoods housed an eclectic mix of churches that competed with each other for believers (*crentes*). On weekends, the streets were filled with the sights and sounds of worship: the beat of drums; the strains of choruses singing in Portuguese, Chitewe, Chisena, Chindau, or any other of the many African languages spoken locally; and the crackle and distortion of amplified sermons projecting beyond the walls of the churches and mosques, mostly constructed of the same humble materials as the homes of the *bairros populares*.

TextÁfrica was once the economic backbone of the city, providing employment to thousands until it closed in 2002.[73] The nonoperational factory stood as testimony to the disappointments of

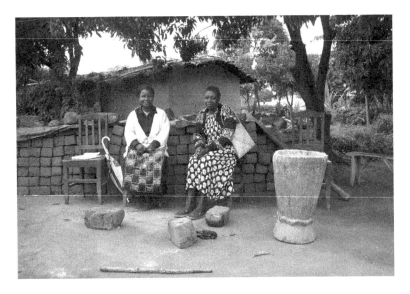

Figure 4. Neighbors posing together in front of a typical *bairro* home.

postcolonial nationhood. The circumstances of TextÁfrica's closure continued to be discussed in Chimoio during my fieldwork. Following trade liberalization mandates of neoliberal economic adjustment, imported Asian textiles and cheap secondhand clothing flooded the local markets, undercutting TextÁfrica's production. Some insisted as well that the factory was mismanaged. Others claimed the factory was intentionally undermined by the independent government because it became a center for political opposition.[74] The overall decline in wage-earning opportunities in the postwar period drove residents into the informal economy. Most Chimoians engaged in a variety of side hustles and odd jobs (*biscate*). These ranged from the selling of small items such as mobile phone credit, home-brewed alcoholic drinks, factory-produced popsicles, and packets of cooking oil to the selling of their labor in construction, security, and domestic work.[75] *Bairro* households combined these side jobs with subsistence production on small plots of land (*machambas*) outside the city. Many participated in cash crop economies, selling tobacco to Zimbabwean and US companies and tomatoes, cabbage, greens, mangos, bananas, and other produce in local markets in and around Chimoio.

FIELDWORK: NEGOTIATING THE AIDS ECONOMY

While I was based in Chimoio, I followed AIDS treatment interventions to smaller towns and rural areas in Manica province. I spent the majority of my time in settings where I could observe AIDS treatment interventions in action, not only in organizations such as associations and Day Hospitals but also in the tight quarters of Chimoio's *bairros*, as well as in smaller towns and rural areas, with people in their homes and churches and on visits to neighbors, relatives, and *n'angas*. I conducted serial semistructured interviews, longitudinally spaced out over time, with over a hundred individuals. I was able to rely on Portuguese for the majority of my interactions, though I also was able to converse in Chitewe and had the help of my field assistant's translations when needed. My longitudinal engagement allowed me to chart the life cycles of organizations and institutions and to attend to the lived experience of a putative global health success story.[76] Throughout my fieldwork, people spoke to me about their experiences, and many opened their lives to me. Some likely held out hope that they would receive some material benefit through my acquaintance, perhaps assuming I had connections and resources, but people also spoke to me and befriended me out of curiosity, novelty, or amusement. My richest data came from many of these informal conversations, interactions, and observations of daily life. I paid particular attention to how local and regional histories influenced contemporary responses to the AIDS epidemic and the treatment scale-up.

I regularly attended meetings of two associations of people living with HIV/AIDS; accompanied community home-based care volunteers from several organizations throughout the region; and interviewed administrators and officials at local, provincial, and national levels. In Chimoio's Day Hospital, I chatted with patients as they waited for appointments, sat in on visits with clinicians and group counseling sessions, and attended clinician meetings. As a medical student at the time, I was not yet practicing medicine, but I was familiar with clinical terminology and the pathophysiology of HIV/ AIDS, so I was able to address many medical questions posed to me by those in treatment regarding HIV/AIDS, antiretroviral side effects, the progress of vaccine research, and how HIV and ARVs impacted fertility.

I worried about how much my own presence, as a *muzungu*, or white person, altered the very dynamics of what I was trying to study. I was often assumed to be a development worker or a missionary. As I began to work in Mozambique, I was concerned that my presence elicited narratives of need that those with HIV/AIDS hoped I might be able to satisfy, and that this would distort what they told me, or worse, that people would feel coerced to talk to me. I was self-conscious about how I would be perceived and how those perceptions would affect the kinds of relationships I was able to form. I was working across significant inequalities based on citizenship, race, and subject position that people regularly pointed out.

This was illustrated during one of my early visits to Mozambique, prior to the ARV scale-up, when an AIDS activist named Suzana introduced me to a support group of HIV positive women. The women were participating in a pilot project designed to demonstrate that ARV treatment was feasible in Mozambique. They were receiving ARVs as well as food for their entire families. Many of the women present said this food helped their families prioritize their treatment and even encouraged some of the women to come forth and seek treatment. Suzana introduced me to the group by declaring: "Do not be scared of talking to this *muzungu*. This *muzungu* is giving you the food you receive here! So if you don't talk to him, he can't help you. He may not have food to give you today, but what you say will travel far, and perhaps it will bring something back." I hastened to correct Suzana, telling the group that I had nothing to do with any food they received, that I was a student on an independent research project, and that I had nothing concrete to offer in exchange for talking to me. After the meeting had ended I asked Suzana to never tell people I was going to give them anything again, lest they be misled or coerced into talking to me in order to receive something.

I often explained I was a student, there to learn and to listen. Many told me they appreciated how patiently I listened. One collaborator who repeatedly told me this, Diogo, who worked in Chimoio's Day Hospital, suggested I put my penchant for listening to use by working in the Day Hospital as a physician once I had finished my research and training. As I developed relationships with people, I contributed to funeral and medical expenses, as well as making gifts of clothing and food. I also was able to contribute my office skills and access to basic office equipment in two associations where I became something of a fixture, contributing to grant applications for organizations whose members had few clerical skills and lacked access to electricity, to say nothing of computers. I was drawn into the kinds of relationships within the AIDS economy that this book addresses: relationships of care and concern, involving reciprocity and exchange across gulfs of knowledge, wealth, and power in a context of widespread poverty and high mortality. Suzana's comment, directed to me as much as it was to the women of the support group, helped me see the high stakes these gradients of inequality created. Her comments reminded me of the multiple ways I was engaging in the AIDS economy, including using the raw material of stories and conversations in the production of my own academic work. Her remarks also emphasized an obligation I had to hear, to understand, and to share these stories.

ORGANIZATION OF THE BOOK

All I Eat Is Medicine is an ethnography of the way a global health treatment intervention became a part of people's everyday lives. It tracks how people took up, adopted, deployed, modified, incorporated, and interrogated the knowledge and practices introduced through AIDS interventions. While *intervention* implies an active entrance or intercession from without or above, *taking up* shifts the locus of agency to social actors themselves, the "target population" of interventions. Global AIDS treatment interventions are conceived, funded, and administered by a variety of institutions, but they are constituted when they are taken up by local actors who are positioned within specific therapeutic and moral economies.

Chapter 1 provides the historical context for the AIDS pandemic and the treatment scale-up. This chapter presents the history of healing in Mozambique as a political and social project of care and inclusion. The colonial and postcolonial history of Mozambique can be read as a struggle for survival by subjects of ruling powers largely oriented toward resource extraction. This context contributes to the devastation of the AIDS epidemic. Much of the AIDS treatment scale-up is shaped by the principles and dynamics of neoliberal governance. Subsequent chapters follow differently positioned individuals through the AIDS economy.

Chapter 2 examines the emergence of an AIDS economy shaped by the implementation of globally circulating treatment interventions in the context of local perspectives on illness and moral economies of care. Amid fears of witchcraft stoked by rising inequality and competition, a treatment that left patients hungry made many suspicious of the true motives and intentions of those providing the treatment. This chapter focuses on the story of Rita and Joaquim, a couple I met through an association of people living with HIV/AIDS. They were both frail when I met them, but their precarious position was belied by their sense of humor. Joaquim usually feigned shock or made chuckling rejoinders as irreverent Rita mocked her husband's pronouncements about life in Mozambique. Their playfulness put me at ease and drew me into their lives, much as their family members and neighbors were similarly drawn to them, and in particular to Rita's charisma. I followed them in and out of the AIDS economy over the course of my research.

Chapters 3, 4, and 5 examine different sites of the AIDS economy. Chapter 3 follows Elena, an AIDS activist and early member of the association of people living with HIV/AIDS, Takashinga ("We Were Brave," in Chitewe). Members of these associations at times resisted and at times embraced the terms of treatment, navigating the tensions between solidarity and the competition for resources that characterized these groups. Within these associations, the notion of *Vida Positiva*, living positively, resonated with evangelical language and practices from local Pentecostal churches. These associations became "therapeutic congregations" that offered forms of care and accompaniment within an individualizing and moralizing frame. Elena introduced me to Arminda, who is the focus of chapter 4. Arminda was one of the founding members of Chimoio's first community home-based care (CHBC) network for people with HIV/AIDS. While Arminda was not HIV positive herself, she cared for scores of neighbors and family members who were as she struggled to improve herself and her community. Despite serving as the foundation of early AIDS outreach and care efforts, Arminda and her colleagues felt they were exploited and abandoned over the course of the AIDS treatment scale-up. Chapter 5 presents the dynamics of care in the Day Hospital. The chapter follows nurse Fátima and her social worker colleagues Pedro and Adélia as they counseled patients, who were required to prove themselves worthy of treatment by meeting a set of biological as well as social criteria that disadvantaged the poorer and less educated.

Chapter 6 considers how AIDS treatment paradoxically exacerbated suffering by addressing a biological condition but not the socioeconomic realities that underlie much of the epidemic's devastation and intractability. Hunger has both a physiological basis and an existential dimension, as talk of hunger expresses an embodied sense of exclusion and disillusionment and points to this ambiguous outcome of ARV treatment. The chapter explores the dynamics of hunger, inequality, and the distribution of food aid within the AIDS economy. The book concludes with a call for a global social medicine that considers the kinds of outcomes highlighted by the subjects of this ethnography, who asked for a more just and transparent distribution of resources and identified issues of livelihood—hunger and unemployment—as their primary concerns.

All I Eat Is Medicine shows how the scale-up of AIDS treatment programs was a complicated process with contradictory and unintended consequences. The focus is on the people at the center of the treatment interventions, not only as patients but also as care providers, activists, and healers as they navigated the AIDS economy, through hunger; clinical programs; NGOs; churches; and the homes of healers, family, neighbors, and friends. They were the target population, the intended recipients of the international community's generosity, idealism, and best efforts. Their stories provide a framework for attending to the inequalities and injustices that people in the treatment programs perceived and experienced, even as their lives were being saved. They also point to many of the dynamic tensions that permeated the treatment programs between the individual and the collective, the visible and the invisible, and scarcity and prosperity. *All I Eat is Medicine* uses the language of hunger, symbolized by a pill that is to be taken twice a day, for a lifetime, to point out connections between individual bodily suffering and biological necessity and social relations and the distribution of material benefits. This book charts the lives of individuals and institutions in the thick of the Mozambican AIDS epidemic during a key moment in Mozambique and global health at the turn of the twenty-first century. It argues that a truly therapeutic intervention for HIV/AIDS treatment must go beyond provision of pills to support inclusive structures of healing and care that account for the material basis for survival and the social basis of health and illness.

1 *Estamos Juntos?*

THE POLITICS OF HEALTH AND SURVIVAL
IN MOZAMBIQUE

Popular understandings of global health and humanitarian intervention often imagine a technology, a treatment, or a form of knowledge traveling from the global north, where it was created and is common, to a tabula rasa, or blank slate, in the global south, where the essential technology neatly fills a preexisting need.[1] In reality, long-standing infrastructures and histories powerfully influence the course of contemporary interventions. An understanding of the way AIDS treatment interventions circulated through and reshaped moral and political economies of care in central Mozambique requires a familiarity with the sedimented histories of care that constitute the terrain upon which the interventions unfolded and that people with HIV/AIDS navigated. Political power, healing, and social belonging are interrelated in Mozambique, where healing is a social and political expression of inclusion and value. The struggle for health has also been a struggle for subsistence, as hunger has played a prominent role in Mozambican history, both as a crisis of survival and an idiom of power. This history of healing as a social and political project provides an important context for understanding contemporary dynamics and discourse around health, hunger, and power in the AIDS economy.

Archaeological evidence and oral tradition indicate that successive Bantu migrations from the Limpopo Valley in the south established sedentary communities in unoccupied territories and displaced or absorbed nomadic bands of hunters and gatherers in the Zimbabwean plateau roughly two thousand years ago.[2] Early groups developed iron-smelting techniques that were used to make hoes for intensive cultivation, and from 850 to 1500 this region was dominated by states that engaged in agricultural activity and raised cattle. They also extracted surface gold and harvested ivory from the local elephant population. The Limpopo and Zambezi Rivers connected wealthy gold-producing regions in the interior to coastal trading networks, and largely autonomous towns along the caravan routes traded with extensive networks of Muslim merchants on the eastern coast of Africa from at least 900.[3] Trade networks may have linked this region to the Mediterranean and Asia as far back as 690.[4]

The well-being of the community was integral to political legitimacy, and local rulers, although not divine themselves, had religious authority, as well as important economic and social responsibilities, as the owners and spiritual guardians of the land. Political power was thus tied to agricultural productivity and the ruler's ability to feed his people.[5] To ensure the health of the people and livestock and the fertility of the fields, the ruler consulted with *n'angas*, who embodied the ancestral spirits to whom the ruler appealed for rain.[6] The divination of *n'angas* was also sought regarding the future possibility of war or famine. These *vadzimu* were the intermediaries between the physical world and a high god. Elaborate religious institutions and rituals reinforced the ruler's position. The health of the community was seen as representing a balance between the natural and spiritual worlds, which intermingled in the daily lives of those in the community. This long-standing entwining of economic, moral, therapeutic, and political power rendered individual and community well-being inseparable from the fertility of the land and livestock and relations with others, including ancestors.

PORTUGUESE COLONIALISM: A POLITICAL ECONOMY OF EXTRACTION

While the Portuguese were initially attracted to the gold and ivory of the African interior, the Indian Ocean location was the linchpin in the global expansion to India and the spice islands of the Portuguese empire. Rather than conquer and control, the Portuguese adapted to local patterns of power and production and in many cases depended on the favor of more powerful local rulers, to whom they paid tribute. But in the late nineteenth and early twentieth centuries, the "Scramble for Africa" increased the intensity of European colonization, channeling Africa's riches into the world economy. Portugal's colonial project in central Mozambique was outsourced to a private concession funded with international capital, the Mozambique Company, which would rule Manica Province from 1890 to 1941. The company used police power to extract taxes and labor for settler plantations and infrastructure projects, purchased agricultural products at depressed prices, and exported African labor to neighboring colonies in exchange for payment. The Company "discarded any pretense of development and transformed its holdings into a massive labor reserve and tax farm from which the company's European and African employees violently extracted peasant surplus."[7] Labor conditions were so aversive that even faced with food shortages, in 1909 people in one district said "they would prefer to eat roots and wild fruits than to [work in] Manica, where they should die."[8]

A report filed in 1925 by American sociologist Edward Ross with the League of Nations's Temporary Slaving Commission highlighted mounting international criticism. Ross quoted a missionary physician's description of the precarious conditions peasants faced: "The chronic state of semi-starvation, in which the majority of people now exist, I attribute to the excessive demands made for labor, leaving insufficient time for the cultivation of their crops." One group of workers told Ross they were "slaves of the Mozambique Company."[9] Regimes of forced labor were continued and refined by the Portuguese administration even after the Mozambique Company's contract expired in 1941.[10] Household labor was diverted from subsistence-level activities to cotton production (demanded for trade and as payment for taxes by Portuguese authorities) to such a degree that food shortages were created. A 1941 survey from the Gaza province in the Limpopo region concluded that "50 percent of the women could not produce the forced cultures without seriously reducing food production."[11] In response to this crisis, cultivation shifted from grain to manioc, which is drought resistant and requires little attention but is significantly less nutritious. Famines were common in the 1940s and 1950s, and a 1959 government report acknowledged: "The majority of the population is underfed," warning that "it is absolutely necessary that cotton producers have sufficient food to enable them to work."[12] The few existing sources of data from hospitals and rural clinics indicate that nutritional diseases, such as kwashiorkor, rickets, scurvy, beriberi, and pellagra, were common.[13]

STRUGGLES FOR SURVIVAL

As colonial conquest created crises of health and survival, prominent *n'angas* responded to safeguard the health and well-being of their communities. Religious leaders and healers helped to legitimize, organize, and coordinate rebellions, uniting public opinion behind uprisings and offering divine sanction and ritual approval of secular leadership.[14] In one uprising in 1902 in Báruè, just northeast of contemporary Chimoio, *n'angas* claimed to have secret medicines that would turn Portuguese bullets into water.[15]

While the Portuguese relationship with indigenous medicine had been characterized by "mutual borrowings for practical healing purposes," the formalization and consolidation of colonial rule in the late nineteenth century marked a change.[16] Colonial biomedicine was deployed as a tool of influence and control over the local population and as propaganda to justify the colonial project internationally.[17] The Portuguese, like other colonial powers, repressed and ruptured local forms of power and knowledge—particularly those of *n'angas*—as these were perceived as threats to colonial authority.[18] Laws were passed against rituals of possession, divination, exorcism, and spiritual healing. Practices related to these activities— drumming, dancing, singing, and prayers directed toward ancestral spirits—were banned as witchcraft. Indigenous healing was relegated to an archaic and irrational African past that was demonized by Christian missions as well as the Portuguese colonial administration. Those caught practicing were imprisoned, sentenced to forced labor, or exiled.[19] Indigenous social and political institutions were co-opted, attacked, and driven underground.

With indigenous healing outlawed, colonial biomedicine took over in countering perceived health threats, predominantly infectious, posed by the native population, with the overarching goal of preserving the labor force and protecting European settlers. The health measures most likely to be experienced by native Mozambicans were restrictions on movement in the name of epidemic containment and forced vaccination and hospitalization.[20] Colonial biomedicine and public health were largely experienced as additional forms of oppression.[21] In Manica and Sofala, the Mozambique Company provided rudimentary health services for its workers. Regarding treatment in the Manica hospital, the company's inspector general noted that "our natives have in some cases been shockingly treated."[22] The director of the native labor department acknowledged that "the native has great repugnance for being treated by whites and much more so for entering the hospital, because they think that once they enter that place they'll never leave. . . . Perhaps there is some logic in their actions because if sometimes they receive good care, at others it leaves a little to be desired."[23] There was no safety net provided for the majority of Mozambicans, and traditional and historical institutions of social cohesion based on agriculture, kinship, and veneration of ancestors were repressed and actively persecuted.[24] Healing was severed from the political order as forms of public healing were driven underground and local clusters of kin had to organize and pay for their own health care in secret within a more circumscribed, private sphere.[25]

As did many African colonies, Mozambique had a bifurcated legal system, called the Indigenato.[26] The Indigenato defined the difference between settler citizen, or *civilizado*, and native subject, *indígena*.[27] It was a form of institutional segregation marked by racial difference.[28] The *civilizado* had full Portuguese citizenship rights and lived under metropolitan civil law, while the *indígena* would live under African law and the particular laws of the individual colonies. This distinction justified coercive labor exploitation and the suppression of native institutions and healing practices in the name of the colonial civilizing mission. Natives could attain the status of the assimilated person (*assimilado*). This third category granted exemption from forced labor as well as some of the benefits of citizenship, though not political participation. It applied to Mozambican and Asian artisans, traders, skilled workers, and long-term urban residents who were able to "civilize themselves," abandon "tribal customs," and live as the settlers did, including converting to Catholicism. The *assimilado* status was also available to those of Asian or mixed racial background. The Indigenato shaped a series of ideological oppositions between native and citizen, traditional and modern, black and white, and rural and urban that endure in contemporary Mozambique and that permeate the logics of HIV/AIDS interventions.

Though the Portuguese justified their colonial presence as first a "civilizing" and then a "modernizing" mission, few Mozambicans ever enjoyed the more powerful political subjectivity of citizenship embodied by the *civilizado*.[29] Amid rising independence and anti-colonial movements, Portugal's effort to justify its ongoing occupation included a post–World War II modernization campaign. This featured large-scale industrialization projects, including textile factories (TextÁfrica in Chimoio, TexLom in Maputo, TexMoque in Nampula) and the Cahora Bassa Dam along the Zambezi River, but what little investment there was in the infrastructure of the colony served the export-oriented priorities of the colonial powers.[30] By 1950 only five thousand Mozambicans out of a population of a few million had become *assimilado*.[31] In 1960 only 10 percent of African Mozambicans were Christian and only 24 percent of Mozambican children attended school. Property and well-paying employment were even more elusive. This almost complete exclusion of native Mozambicans from the benefits of citizenship constituted one of the central platforms of the liberation movements that emerged during the late 1950s and culminated in the formation of the Front for the Liberation of Mozambique (Frente de Libertação de Moçambique; Frelimo).

Frelimo was led by black Mozambican intellectuals who had attended mission schools and often had received foreign education. Frelimo initiated a guerrilla war in 1964, operating from bases in Tanzania and then within Mozambique from "liberated villages" under its control. Portuguese counterinsurgency tactics included massacres and forced resettlement of peasants to government-built villages under military surveillance, ostensibly to protect them from anti-colonial guerrillas.[32] These villages (*aldeamentos*), with improved facilities for health care and education as well as infrastructural developments in water provision and agriculture, were attempts to not only cut off the rebels from their bases of support but to "win the hearts and minds of Africans through modernizing development."[33] This was paired with increasingly brutal military tactics in the early 1970s that involved the use of napalm exfoliants and ongoing massacres of villages suspected of harboring Frelimo guerrillas. Frelimo, on the other hand, emphasized education in its liberated zones, creating "a vast network of bush-based elementary schools." Children and adults learned to read and write in Portuguese and studied mathematics and the natural sciences in order to administer the agricultural cooperatives and health posts that Frelimo established.[34] Eventually the expense of Portugal's wars across its colonial empire in terms of resources and human lives (one in four adult Portuguese males were being conscripted for the African wars) contributed to a coup d'état in Portugal 1974.[35] Mozambique would gain independence in 1975.

INDEPENDENCE, SOVEREIGNTY, AND HEALTH

Lack of public services under colonialism had been one of the chief complaints of the national liberation movement, and the provision of medical services and education was a top concern of the independent government.[36] Samora Machel, a former nurse and the first president of Mozambique, declared: "The hospital is the only contact many people have with the state. It touches their most sensitive point: health, well-being, and their very life."[37] At independence, Mozambique's under-age-five mortality approached 25 percent, and there was one African among the 519 doctors in Mozambique, a number that dwindled to 86 after independence.[38] Ninety-five percent of Mozambicans were illiterate.[39] Providing their citizens basic health and education services was a cornerstone of Frelimo's economic program and the basis of the new government's legitimacy (see figure 5). A vaccination campaign in the first years of independence covered 95 percent of the population, which at that time was a world record. All health care was nationalized in 1977 when the NHS was established, under which services were made effectively free and a primary health care approach was adopted. Forty-five hundred

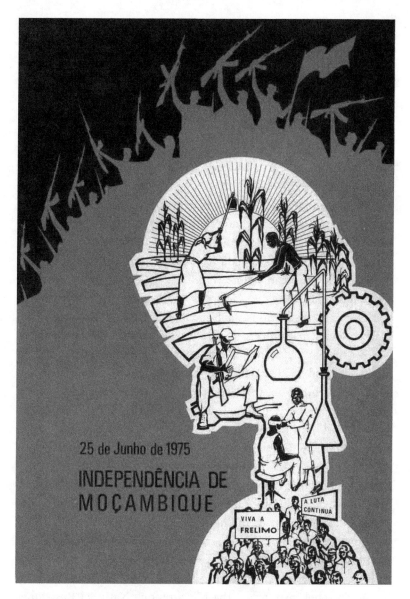

Figure 5. Poster celebrating the pillars of Mozambican independence: agricultural labor, education, science and industry, health care, and urban mobilization. Design by José Freire, DNPP (Mozambique, 1975), IISH call nr: BG E9/737.

health workers were trained by 1982, one hundred of whom were doctors. The number of health posts increased from 326 at independence to 1,122 in 1983.[40] Pharmaceutical import costs were reduced by 40 percent via competitive bidding from foreign suppliers on basic drugs. The World Bank concluded that "since independence Mozambique has been in the vanguard in the development of broadbased primary health care and in the implementation of an essential drugs program. . . . Mozambique has done much better than other African countries."[41]

Frelimo's emphasis on basic services brought it domestic support, and its progressive policies and promotion of comprehensive primary care and education and women's rights were popular internationally. But the ambitious agenda to create a new Mozambique based on "scientific socialism" ironically led to the perpetuation of oppressive colonial practices and ideologies.[42] Frelimo attacked traditional authority and institutions for impeding progress.[43] It campaigned against social institutions such as bride wealth (dowries paid to families for the loss of the productive and reproductive labor of their daughters) and tried to undermine traditional hierarchies based on power differentials between elders and youth and men and women. Widespread property nationalization created dissidents among the affluent, as did the forced relocation of private farmers to state farms, all too reminiscent of the Portuguese *aldeamentos*. *N'angas*, considered purveyors of backward superstition, were also forbidden to practice (a stance that Frelimo reversed in 1992, establishing the National Association of Traditional Healers, Associação de Médicos Tradicionais de Moçambique or AMETRAMO).

The country's apartheid neighbors, Southern Rhodesia and South Africa, also stoked resentment among Mozambicans who felt marginalized from or opposed to Frelimo's revolutionary project. In 1976 a rebel insurgency, the Mozambique National Resistance (Resistência Nacional Moçambicano; Renamo), was organized by Rhodesian security forces to target anti-apartheid groups based in

Mozambique who were fighting for African independence in Rhodesia.[44] Renamo's early recruits were from the black military and paramilitary groups who had fought for the Portuguese. While the official US State Department stance toward Renamo was critical, the Central Intelligence Agency was supportive, as was "a frightful laundry list of right-wing American sects and organizations," which characterized the Renamo insurgents as "freedom fighters" and sent aid through a "ramshackle system of privatized intervention."[45] But rather than articulating a cohesive alternative to Frelimo's government, Renamo's mission was to destabilize the fledgling nation. The resulting civil war between Frelimo and Renamo is recognized as one of the bloodiest and most devastating conflicts of the twentieth century.

In the sixteen years of war, one million people, the majority noncombatants and half of these children, lost their lives. Half of the national population of sixteen million was directly affected by the war and may have been subjected to "attack, rape, torture, forced relocation, kidnapping, and forced servitude at an army base."[46] Many were forced to witness atrocities and participate in violence, and one-fourth of the population fled their homes. Over one-third of schools and clinics were destroyed or closed. Roads were rendered impassable due to attacks or land mines.[47]

Destabilization disrupted trade and led to rising prices, black markets, and shortages in basic commodities, provoking an economic crisis for Frelimo. A severe drought in 1982 took 100,000 lives. Out of a desperate desire for emergency aid, Frelimo initiated discussions with Western donors. In exchange for food aid and drought relief in 1983, donors required Mozambique to fundamentally restructure economic and social policy. This led to a political-economic about-face as Mozambique transitioned from a centrally planned socialist economy to Western privatization, deregulation, and free markets. The objectives of Mozambique's apartheid neighbors to incapacitate the socialist government were thus met, as the country was left as "the world's poorest, hungriest, most indebted, most aid-dependent country."[48]

CHRISTIANITY, SALVATION, AND POWER

As a part of its "scientific socialism" agenda, Frelimo dismissed religion, nationalized religious schools, and excluded Christians from party membership. Some denominations were persecuted and their members deported or sent to reeducation camps.[49] This occurred despite the fact that many Frelimo leaders were mission educated. Frelimo justified this policy by citing the long-standing collaboration between Catholicism and colonialism. Samora Machel is said to have declared that "the Catholic church was the church of the colonial fascist regime."[50] Indeed, the Catholic church was often instrumentalized by the Portuguese to support their political influence and was a key component of the earliest Portuguese presence in East Africa in the sixteenth century.

The scramble for Africa at the turn of the twentieth century brought Portugal rivals in spiritual as well as political and economic domains. International treaties allowed all religious missions to work in countries of their choice, bringing Protestant missions into Mozambique in the 1880s. In 1940 the Portuguese state had granted the Catholic church the exclusive right to educate Africans, but schooling only advanced to the second grade, and in some urban areas to the fourth grade. Local languages were taboo, and no Africans were trained to be teachers. One of Frelimo's early leaders, Eduardo Mondlane, characterized the Catholic church's education efforts as aimed at preparing a subservient workforce and perpetuating Africans' status as second-class citizens.[51] The mainline Protestant missions were openly critical of the Catholic notion of civilization, and they emphasized local languages and informal systems of education relying on youth, laity, and communities.[52] They served as a nucleus of Mozambican nationalism and opposition to colonialism, educating many of the eventual leaders and professional class of the independence movement, including Eduardo Mondlane and Samora Machel.[53]

In addition to Catholicism and the Protestant missions, a third strand of Christianity was imported in the early twentieth century

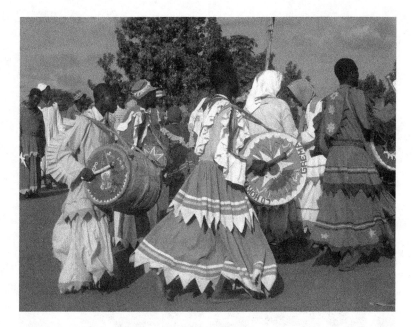

Figure 6. African Independent Church service.

via migrant laborers exposed to "Apostolic Faith" and "Zionist" evangelists in South Africa and Southern Rhodesia. They returned to Mozambique as converts, preachers, and evangelists of the African Independent Churches (AICs), indigenous churches led by Africans. An observer in the southern province of Inhambane noted that as these workers returned from the neighboring colonies with newfound economic power, these Christian evangelists took over chiefly roles, such as holding seed-sowing ceremonies and dispensing medicine and justice.[54] AICs were at times called "traditional" or "spiritualist" churches because they integrated some aspects of traditional African beliefs and practices into Christian doctrine and worship, including the use of drums in their prayer services (see figure 6), for example, or the tolerance of polygamy. In particular, these churches featured strong syncretic healing practices embodied in the figure of the *profete* (see figure 7). Much like Catholic and Protestant missions,

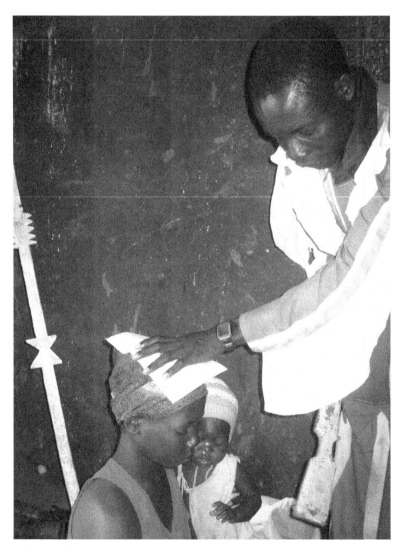

Figure 7. Profete lays hands on a patient as part of a faith-healing ritual.

however, the AICs denigrated the *n'anga*. Despite Portugal's opposition and overt oppression, these churches took root and spread through clandestine forms of door-to-door evangelism.[55] They are today considered to be the earliest African Pentecostal churches.[56]

NEOLIBERAL REFORM AND
THE PENTECOSTAL EXPLOSION

By the mid-1980s, the conflict had left the government deeply in debt, prompting desperate measures. In 1985 Frelimo urged its members to buy private property as a way of contributing to the economy, and in 1986 Mozambique agreed to an Economic Rehabilitation Program (Programa de Reabilitação Econômica; PRE), a World Bank/International Monetary Fund–sponsored structural adjustment program.[57] The program mandated immediate austerity, including government budget cuts to health and social safety nets, market deregulation, aggressive debt repayment, and privatization of many national resources.[58] Within a year of the PRE, the monthly minimum wage fell from $52 to $23.[59] In 1988, half of the urban and two-thirds of the rural population were "absolutely" poor.[60]

The violence of the war that lasted from 1977 to 1992 displaced 40 percent of Mozambicans and destroyed transportation, education, communication, and health infrastructure. Renamo particularly targeted the NHS, attacking primary health care clinics, kidnapping and killing health workers, and overall severely disrupting the health services and preventive programs that the Frelimo government prioritized.[61] Despite this onslaught, the system persisted in providing services. Structural adjustment program caps on NHS budgets, however, effectively prevented the revitalization of the postwar health system. Following the cease-fire in 1995, the health sector was propped up largely through international donor funds funneled to NGOs, with individual provinces being assigned to different national development groups. The United Nations and scores of international relief agencies and NGOs flooded the country to assist with the reconstruction effort. The international "militants who share a common cause" (*cooperantes*) of the independence era, who had worked in the health sector on government contracts, were replaced by the humanitarian aid workers, employees, and consultants from international NGOs.[62] The combined effects of the war and structural adjustment resulted in limited access to basic health care at a critical juncture in the AIDS epidemic.[63] The number of health centers remains below the prewar levels of the late 1970s.[64]

After Frelimo legalized NGOs and religious expression following the civil war, borders opened, traffic increased, and populations moved back and forth. These circumstances allowed Pentecostal proselytizers to establish new churches, just as HIV was following these same roads into Mozambique.[65] A new wave of Pentecostalism brought the influence of born-again, Pentecostal Charismatic Christianity (PCC), which emerged globally in the 1970s, alongside the still-popular AICs. Like the AICs, PCC churches incorporate strict codes of personal ethics; a belief in the imminent second coming of Jesus; and a belief in the "gifts of the spirit," including glossolalia (speaking in tongues), prophecy, faith healing, and exorcism.[66] Important differences exist between the AICs and the born-again PCC churches, however. The PCC churches are more often linked to transnational networks, such as the Brazilian Universal Church of the Kingdom of God. PCC pastors, like those of mission churches and mainstream Protestant and Catholic clergy, tend to have more formal theological training than AIC pastors. While the AICs disdain worldliness and wealth, PCC churches preach a "prosperity gospel," which teaches that God blesses the faithful with material prosperity. AICs tend to appeal to the poorest, while international PCC targets the upwardly mobile working class and aspiring professionals. On the other hand, the Catholic church tends to appeal to the middle class and elite, while the mainline Protestant faiths are most popular among well-educated urban residents.

In Mozambique, PCC church leaders disdained the "backwardness" represented by the AICs and did not consider them to be truly Christian. The *profetes* were seen as equivalent to *n'angas*. In practice, however, it could be difficult to identify the lineages of individual churches, particularly as they usually combined aspects of various denominations. In my conversations with pastors about these distinctions, they often pointed out which of the aspects of Pentecostalism their churches embraced and which they did not. A group of churches called Zion Pentecostal explicitly tried to combine AIC and PCC principles. One pastor described his church as being "part Zionist, part Assembly of God"—that is, part regionally grounded AIC, part cosmopolitan, globally connected Pentecostal.[67] Due to the widespread popularity of *profetes*, even international Pentecostals have begun prophet healing, and while PCC churches embrace spiritual healing, they do not believe this needs to be performed by a *profete*, arguing that it is God that heals, and this healing can happen through pastors or even church members, often through a laying on of hands. Despite this concession, the PCC disdain for "tradition" offers a radical break from "African superstition" and an appealing link to modernity and the material world beyond Mozambique.[68]

The post–civil war explosion in church activity coincided with the rise of a conspicuous culture of international development, represented by SUVs emblazoned with organizational logos and bustling enclaves of expatriates and well-to-do Mozambicans.[69] The development sector includes a heterogeneous mix of large transnational donors; smaller transnational, national, and regional NGOs; and their local partners. Many Mozambicans pointed to the emergence of churches and NGOs as among the defining characteristics of postwar life, and the ways these spheres interacted significantly shaped the dynamics of the AIDS economy that emerged with the treatment scale-up.

PEACE WITHOUT BENEFIT

Enthusiastic political engagement and an egalitarian spirit balanced the austerity of the early independence period. There was great optimism and hope for a new social structure based on equality and self-determination. "We are together" (*estamos juntos*) became a popular slogan of solidarity that has endured to the present day. Food was rationed through state-run "people's shops" and neighborhood-based consumer cooperatives. Basic staples were subsidized, and households were issued monthly ration cards. Health and education were universally available, free of charge until structural adjustment–mandated strangulation of the public sector led to official and unofficial user fees. During my research, many expressed nostalgia for the revolutionary period. A motorist employed by an NGO who had worked for the NHS in the early years of independence recalled that prices were low and nearly everyone was employed. Volunteers were granted perks, like the first chance to buy from state consumer cooperatives. As the war progressed and the economy collapsed, however, the shelves of the cooperatives were bare and people waited in line for hours for bread. Now, he noted, there were many shops with shelves full of goods, but few could afford to buy anything in them. While many had volunteered during the revolutionary period, rising costs of living and fewer public supports now made volunteering difficult.

Mozambican sociologist Elísio Macamo argues that with the turn to neoliberalism there was a fundamental shift in Frelimo's ideology. Mozambique's newly independent government idealized "serving the people," and politicians were subjected to a strict moral code that was influenced by not only a Marxist ideology but also the strong Protestant background of many of Frelimo's leaders. Observers of the era claimed there was little corruption.[70] During the revolution, the antithesis of the "revolutionary man" of scientific socialism was a slovenly, pot-bellied cartoon character named "Xiconhoca," whose selfishness and dubious moral conduct risked undermining the entire project of social transformation. Structural adjustment reforms, on the other hand, gave legitimacy to individualism while simultaneously rolling back the state, increasing pressure on social networks of kin and religion.[71] Frelimo removed references to socialism from the constitution and national anthem, and the everyday discourse of government officials touted the advantages offered by private investment, free trade, the virtues of the market, and the benefits of competition.[72]

HUNGER, HEALTH, AND ECONOMIC GROWTH

Portuguese colonialism in the twentieth century exacerbated the historical challenges of scarcity and hunger in the region and provoked a large-scale crisis of health and survival whose repercussions continue to reverberate. Indigenous institutions for healing and social cohesion were systematically repressed, while basic survival was threatened by a regime of ruthless extraction. Hunger has been a prominent aspect of both lived experience and political critique in Mozambique for at least the past century. At independence, there was widespread hope that the revolutionary Frelimo government would fulfill its promises to redress the historic disenfranchisement of the majority of the population by specifically prioritizing health and livelihood, but the deliberate destruction of infrastructure and the rising toll of human lives during the civil war impeded and reversed much of the progress in this direction. With the end of the civil war in 1992, donor prescriptions to foster "civil society" resulted in burgeoning inequality and profound disappointment.

A 2007 World Bank report that proclaimed Mozambique a success on the strength of a "blistering pace of economic growth" also reported a "paradox": as gross domestic product (GDP) continued to grow, child malnutrition increased as well.[73] Development scholar and longtime observer of Mozambique Joseph Hanlon's review of the World Bank report noted that living standards were insecure and that quantitative reductions in poverty were exaggerated, as they failed to account for the fact that people were eating more low-nutrition manioc for economic reasons, leading to more malnutrition.[74] Indeed, half the population suffered from malnutrition.[75]

In 2016 the IMF warned: "In Mozambique, income inequality has increased despite high rates of economic growth"; "few countries offer such a stark contrast as Mozambique. Benefits of growth have not been broadly shared and high levels of inequality hamper government policies to reduce poverty."[76] The neoliberal World Bank/IMF model assumes that people will earn enough money to survive through self-employment and the informal sector. However, the majority of poor people lacked the assets to access the market-centered model and thus could not pull themselves out of poverty.

In the late 1960s Eduardo Mondlane wrote about the importance of equality while articulating Frelimo's early vision of governance: "The biggest danger is the formation of new groups of privileged Africans. Paradoxically, to block the concentration of wealth and services in small areas of the country in the hands of few, strong central planning is necessary."[77] Nearly forty years later, Armando Guebuza, president during the AIDS treatment scale-up of the mid-2000s, embodied the move away from this position as he became one of the richest men in the country during the economic transition away from socialism.[78] Addressing a crowd in central Mozambique, Guebuza proclaimed "it makes no sense that in a country with plenty of fertile land and major rivers there should be so many people with nothing to eat, and living in dire poverty." Guebuza insisted that if Mozambicans were willing to work hard, they would do away with poverty, insisting poverty and hunger existed because of the lack of "a habit and love for work."[79] The structural adjustment programs that accompanied aid from the World Bank and the IMF exported such precepts to much of the global south, pushing the idea that in order to thrive, people must take responsibility for themselves and work hard to take advantage of opportunities, and that a failure to do so represents a personal, moral, and ethical failing. This racialized discourse echoed colonial notions that Mozambicans needed to be "civilized" and taught to work.[80] Hanlon argues that "the whole aid industry is predicated on the nineteenth century view that rich people should come in to train the poor and force them to behave properly."[81] In other words, such approaches assume that the poor are responsible for their own poverty and hunger.

Guebuza's call for autonomy and self-responsibility was a departure from both revolutionary Frelimo and the notions of personhood that have existed in the region from the precolonial period. Historically, personhood in southeastern Africa has been understood as constituted through pro-social relationships with others and through mutuality, reciprocation, and ethics of interdependence. In this context, Guebuza's statement sounds radically individualistic. Neoliberalism is the outcome of a capitalist, individualist worldview; it presents a particular vision of the relationship between individuals, markets, and the state that some have described as "the death of the social."[82] Into this new Mozambican world—one that had turned from *estamos juntos* to neoliberal individualism, in which the majority suffered under the market-centered model rather than being elevated by it, ravaged by four hundred years of colonial extraction, a devastating apartheid-sponsored civil war, a long history of hunger, the undermining of biomedical and social infrastructure, the repression of indigenous traditions of healing and health care, and the entrenchment of deep poverty—the disease of the century arrived. A global network of activists, interventions, pharmaceuticals, NGOs, and policy frameworks would follow, spawning the AIDS economy.

2 The Emergence of the AIDS Economy

We heard about a serious disease, coming from far
away, not here. When it arrived, it did so quietly, it
was hidden, no one knew. People had it, were going
to the hospital, but we didn't know, nobody knew.
It was all in secret. These VCTs, ARVs, these are
new, they just arrived.

Rita

Rita lived with her husband, Joaquim, in a two-room hut on a small
lot bordered by train tracks on one side in a *bairro popular* in Chimoio's cane city. The roar of a passing engine occasionally inter-
rupted our conversations when I visited. Rita tested positive in
late 2004 at a voluntary counseling and testing center (VCT) and
would start ARVs within the year. The infrastructure that made
the illness visible and provided her with treatment had only just
materialized. Prior to the availability of testing and treatment, Rita
recalled, AIDS appeared to be a rumor. She had lost three of her
four pregnancies with Joaquim, and "everything hurt, headaches,
stomach, the whole body, there was not one spot that was well." She
attributed this to a spirit that possessed her: "I would go to *n'anga*,
they'd say I was possessed by a spirit. We didn't know anything, just
of spirits, that's all."

Rita decided to get tested at the encouragement of her sister's husband. He belonged to an association of people living with HIV/ AIDS. He revealed to her that he was HIV positive himself and that he recognized some of the same signs in her that he had experienced. He advised her to get tested and to join the association if she turned out to be positive. Many were introduced to the illness in this way, by trusted kin. Joaquim would eventually test positive as well, and both would start ARVs. Both would continue to seek treatment from healers for spiritual ailments.

At the start of the AIDS treatment scale-up, HIV/AIDS was interpreted through existing frameworks of health and illness in Mozambique, which were broader and more grounded in social relationships than in biomedical understandings. Despite what clinical personnel and AIDS educators often asserted, diagnosis and treatment were not straightforward matters of knowledge versus ignorance, a binary echoing the colonial dualisms of *civilizado* versus *indígena* and modernity versus tradition. Rita and Joaquim drew on a relational economy of care in which good health depended upon good relationships with neighbors and kin. Cultivating and maintaining such relationships entailed maintaining ties of reciprocity and obligation. Health in the AIDS economy, however, according to the precepts of *Vida Positiva*—living positively—was framed in terms of individual agency, knowledge, and responsibility rather than in terms of relationship, reciprocity, and obligation, a shift in values and norms reflecting neoliberal reforms. An entrepreneurial hustle surrounded AIDS treatment programs. The move "from fear to hope" proved to be a part of an increasingly competitive sector and at times another sphere of marginalization.[1] In this way, illness, inequality, and treatment interventions came together to create a neoliberal AIDS economy in central Mozambique that intensified exclusion, suspicion, and hunger. The norms, responsibilities, and assumptions of this neoliberal AIDS economy came into conflict with the locally grounded relational economy of care.

NAVIGATING THE THERAPEUTIC ECONOMY

Multiple, often contradictory ethical imperatives, modes of diagnosis and treatment, and caregiving obligations comprised
Mozambique's "therapeutic economy," a concept developed by
physician-anthropologist Vinh-Kim Nguyen in his work on AIDS
in West Africa. The concept is based on "the totality of therapeutic
options in a given location, as well as the rationale underlying the
patterns of resort by which these therapies are accessed."[2] Joaquim
had been well until one day the previous month when he fainted
after he'd been carrying a heavy load. He suspected witchcraft
because the onset of his illness was sudden, right after seeing a flash
of light as he was resting in his *quintal* at home. He soon began running a high fever, sweating profusely, and vomiting. He was certain
he was suffering the effects of an *espírito mau*, sent by someone with
malicious intent. Even though he knew he had tested positive before,
he reasoned that HIV "affects you little by little, not all of a sudden."
Rita interjected to contribute to his explanation: "Our problem here
is witchcraft, envy." The tight quarters of Chimoio's congested living
conditions and competition for resources between strangers as well
as kin exacerbated anxieties about malice, envy, and witchcraft. In
precolonial times, this envy might have been of a neighbor's bounti-
ful harvest. In contemporary Mozambique, it could be envy of store-
bought clothes or a cash-paying job.[3] Rita explained the difference:
"If it's a problem from God, we run to the hospital. But when it's
something that someone did, you've got to first go address that [by
going to a *n'anga* or *profete*]."

People who were HIV positive were also understood to be more
vulnerable to witchcraft. Joaquim explained that this risk itself was
a reason to keep the diagnosis secret:

> People say, "oh, that person was already sick with AIDS and that's
> what killed him," while it was actually another person who did it.
> Nobody would know. So when you get sick, you always have to look

into these things. But it must be hidden when someone asks you how you are feeling. You can't just say I'm taking antiretrovirals, because if you tell everything, another person can take advantage, send things, and you could die.

Joaquim continued, pointing out that the *espírito mau* causing the illness also could affect hospital staff and the entire clinical apparatus: "It closes those people, and you do not even look human to them. The tests won't come out correctly." If "complicated" spiritual diseases are left untreated, the spiritual agents can cloud and distort the judgment of the sick individual or the providers, or even the validity of clinical instruments and tests. I encountered this as a frequent explanation of why individuals often sought spiritual therapy before or at the same time as biomedical care.

While biomedicine could diagnose and effectively intervene in "natural" illnesses, its focus on the individual body did not speak to social reality. African healing practitioners understand most diseases to have a relational origin. HIV/AIDS occupied an ambiguous space in the "natural" versus "relational" binary. It was diagnosed and treated by biomedicine, which did not recognize "relational" diseases. While some sexually transmitted diseases were understood to be "natural"— *zwirwere zwemunjanji* (literally diseases from the railway, so named because migrant workers brought them home when they returned from the Rhodesian mines) or *zvirwere zvepabonde* (diseases from the sleeping mat)—and to require medicinal remedy, others, like *piringaniso*, were linked to immoral sexual activity and understood to be "relational."[4] The reported symptoms of *piringaniso*—loss of strength (*kupera simba*), loss of appetite (*kusada kudya*), nausea (*kushotwa*), and fever (*kupisa mwiri*, literally hot body)—also match AIDS symptoms. Unlike other sexually transmitted diseases, both "natural" and "relational," HIV/AIDS stood out as one of the few diseases to not have a cure and to inevitably lead to death. In regional healing paradigms, death is associated with the withdrawal of ancestral protection or witchcraft. It is never "natural."[5]

N'angas attributed at least part of the perceived morbidity of the AIDS epidemic to the fact that people were no longer observing traditions, particularly in urban areas. There was also some disagreement about whether *piringaniso* and HIV/AIDS were just similar conditions or whether one was mistaken for the other.[6] One elder *n'anga* who had been practicing since 1960 spoke of a convergence of HIV and *piringaniso*: "When I began working as a *n'anga*, the disease HIV/AIDS did not exist. We did have this disease *piringaniso*, however. Over the years, these diseases have come together. Now [people say], we don't see *piringaniso*, we see AIDS. *Piringaniso* still exists! But someone with *piringaniso* goes to the test, they say it's AIDS, but the problem is *piringaniso*." This sentiment spoke to the long-standing mistrust of the state by *n'angas*, resulting from the history of state antagonism toward healers as backward *indígena*, mired in African tradition and ignorant of the modern biomedicine of the *civilizado*.[7]

N'angas and *profetes* might disagree regarding the diagnosis or the necessary course of action in individual cases, and they were wary of always accepting the authority of biomedicine, but most did not deny the existence of HIV. They participated in HIV/AIDS trainings sponsored by the Ministry of Health (Ministério da Saúde; MISAU). They were eager to learn about this new illness and even asked for more responsibilities in the effort, such as the ability to test their patients for HIV. *N'angas* and *profetes* also sent their patients to clinics and hospitals at times, but they were generally blamed for delaying biomedical treatment. Most who worked in the AIDS treatment interventions denigrated healers for these delays and for propagating misinformation about HIV/AIDS. Churches, particularly those that were mainstream Protestant and Pentecostal, similarly dismissed *n'angas* as pagan relics of the past. *N'angas*, however, attributed the rising popularity of the churches as part of the abandonment of tradition that gave rise to spiritual afflictions.

Official AIDS education efforts seemed to have added to the alienation of those who saw themselves as guardians of tradition and morality, as "sex positive" messages and hip, suggestive condom marketing campaigns enraged elders and religious leaders, who accused the government and development organizations of encouraging prostitution. Public educational demonstrations of condom use were seen as disrespectful, emblematic of a young generation that no longer respected the old.[8]

When illness was understood to be "relational," quests for treatment were shaped by suspicions of external threat and malice as well as material constraint. Illness brought up the question not only of "what is happening to me" but also of "who has done this to me." Witchcraft is a feature of settings in which "competition pits individualism and communalism against each other."[9] AIDS emerged in environments already swirling with these fears of sent sickness.[10] In a context where individual agency was significantly constrained by broader social and material forces, knowledge of HIV serostatus was only one factor dictating how and when treatment was sought. Social and material support was of crucial significance and often dictated diagnosis and treatment.[11] For these reasons, despite Rita's urging, Joaquim would not to return to the Day Hospital even after a positive diagnosis and recurrence of illness.

THE SOCIAL MEANING OF WITCHCRAFT: TERESA'S STORY

Teresa, who lived in a neighborhood just a fifteen-minute walk from the hospital, was also worried about her vulnerability to *uroi*, despite living with HIV and despite encouragement from friends to seek treatment in the Day Hospital. One of her neighbors invited me to accompany him on a visit to Teresa one Sunday morning before he went to church. Teresa's older brother chatted with us while a young boy told Teresa she had visitors. The boy returned and led us through a narrow doorway, whereupon we entered the dark, cramped room where Teresa lay on a straw mat under a coarse woolen blanket. Next to Teresa sat her elderly mother in her brightly patterned *capulana*, with a baby tightly wrapped to her back.[12]

It was a blustery June morning, and I was glad to join Teresa and her mother next to a cluster of glowing coals underneath a small, iron stove with a bubbling pot on top. We sat on wooden stools that Teresa's mother provided, and Teresa sat up and turned to face us. She was frail and slight, and she coughed frequently. Occasionally a gust of wind blew the door open, loudly fluttering and snapping the black tarp stretched across bamboo that served as the roof. Each time, Teresa would stop talking and glare at the door from across the room. Her mother would hastily shut it, even using a rock as a doorstop, but the frame was not well attached to the wall, and it shook with each gust, eventually creaking the door back open. The hard rains of the previous season had taken their toll on many such houses in Chimoio, and it would take time before the family could scrape together the resources to make repairs.

Teresa's neighbor pointed to a cup of a thick mixture next to Teresa, asking: "Is this the treatment you are taking?" Teresa explained it was an herbal mixture from a *n'anga*. Teresa had also been to the Day Hospital, but she was frustrated by the long lines and the lack of treatment she received there. Her husband took her to a *n'anga*, who told her "people in your husband's house have treated you," indicating *uroi* (see figure 8). Teresa was her husband's second wife, and she suspected her co-wife had sent this sickness. Teresa left her husband's house and returned to stay with her own natal family, where she felt safer. Her husband continued to support her, however, and to seek a remedy with her. Relational illnesses point to social ruptures that need to be repaired, often by bringing together the aggrieved parties and by reinforcing social rules. This is frequently accomplished through ritual means. Teresa's diagnosis pointed to a distinct social etiology that made sense to her and her husband given the context within which she fell ill, a conflict with her co-wife. For Teresa, the treatment with the *n'anga* was an opportunity to restore her place in her husband's house. He would speak to his first wife about the

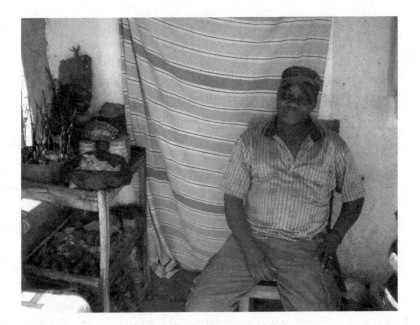

Figure 8. N'anga at his market stall with herbal medications.

incident and try to broker a truce, as the *n'anga* treated Teresa and the entire household. It is not likely an HIV diagnosis would engender the same response from Teresa's husband. He might wonder where she got it from and suspect her of infidelity, since he was not sick himself. The *n'anga's* diagnoses offered a meaningful explanation of the illness, embedded within kin relations, and gave Teresa and her family hope.

The changes over recent decades in central Mozambique increased social and economic vulnerability for many people in the central region, especially women like Teresa.[13] Historically, families in the region lived in large, extended, multigenerational, patrilocal, and frequently polygynous, rurally dispersed household compounds.[14] Contemporary urban settlements were more likely to be nuclear, single- or two-generation households, thus decreasing the availability of kin-based support systems. Following the national transition to a free market economy and a reduction of social protections, cash income became increasingly crucial to survival. This put women at a disadvantage, as they had fewer opportunities for earning cash and earned far less than men.[15] With women more dependent upon their male spouses and relatives for cash, the kind of health care they could access was dependent on the approval of those with expendable cash, such as in Teresa's case. Cash was a necessity for many kinds of therapy. The implementation of fees for public biomedical services and the unofficial additional fees often solicited, as well as hikes in the *n'anga* fees in Chimoio, account for at least some of the popularity of *profetes*, who tended to charge less for their services.[16] The "free market" model for therapeutic services put considerable strain on the poor, who bear the highest burden of disease, and on women.

AIDS activists and treatment providers often spoke of treatment seeking in terms of choices that assumed fealty to a particular therapeutic paradigm, denigrating treatment by *n'angas* and *profete* as obstacles to timely treatment. But the process of responding to illness and misfortune was pragmatic and involved the mobilization of social ties as well as a trying out of different ideas, making and revising plans, and attempting different rituals and techniques.[17] The accounts of Teresa and Rita and Joaquim reveal that there were multiple therapeutic options available, yet few were readily trusted or easily accessible. Many with HIV/AIDS pursued a variety of treatment options until they obtained the results they desired.

"AIDS KILLS": THE STAKES OF VISIBILITY

Given the scale of disruption and suffering caused by the war, the destruction of the health-care infrastructure, and the inability to diagnose and treat HIV/AIDS, perhaps it is no surprise that during the early years of the epidemic many like Rita perceived AIDS as a distant and theoretical threat, as a rumor. Over the course of my fieldwork, many people living with HIV/AIDS recalled how they first learned of AIDS. Suraia, a lively and outspoken member of the same association of people living with HIV/AIDS that Rita and Joaquim belonged to, remembered first learning about AIDS in the early 1990s while watching Zimbabwean television:

> We'd hear that there existed this disease that has no cure. It showed African countries, people dying of what? This illness. Then as each year passed, you'd hear that, here in Mozambique, some people, you never heard how many, but that some people were affected.

Others, like Nanci, a shy woman in her early twenties, recalled first having heard of AIDS just a few years prior, but never paying much attention. Until she herself had the diagnosis, "I didn't believe it existed, I thought it was a lie." Luiz, about whom we'll hear more in Chapter 3, had recently regained his health and his ability to work, saying, "I only really believed it was real when I was losing friends. Then I got sick. It was the same disease, I said to myself, that one they've been talking about. It exists."

The initial mass media campaigns addressing AIDS in Mozambique relied on fatalistic metaphors associating AIDS with death, such as "AIDS Kills!" (*SIDA Mata!*) and "Think of life! Avoid AIDS!" (*Pense na vida! Evite SIDA!*).[18] These messages were propagated via television, radio, posters and billboards, and public presentations (*palestras*). I encountered a poster version of this type of campaign that was produced in the 1990s and featured captioned quotations beneath pictures of national figures.[19] Then president Joaquim Chissano's caption read: "In our young country, we should do everything possible to not succumb as a people and as a nation. The fight against AIDS is the task of each of us." The association of AIDS with catastrophe and chaos, a threat to the integrity of the fragile young country, provided a continuity with the recently ended civil war and framed a "fight" against AIDS as a patriotic duty and an individual responsibility.

The repertoire of representations, concepts, and stereotypes associated with AIDS both reflected and shaped popular beliefs. Another national politician intoned: "Prostitution is the main distributor of this affliction." A religious leader added: "The carriers of HIV should face the reality and in good faith not transmit to others." And a dancer asked: "Even if a cure is found for AIDS, how much will it cost our country?" The suggestion that prostitution was to blame for the illness mobilized colonial and postcolonial tropes of a pathologized and immoral female sexuality. The statements betrayed a fear of the HIV positive while positioning the prevention of transmission as an individual moral and civic duty. The only mention of treatment was fatalistic, emphasizing the lack of a cure and the assumption that were one to be developed, the cost would be prohibitive. As in other contexts, the threat of AIDS was projected onto dangerous and immoral "others."[20] One conspicuously absent voice was that of those who were living with HIV/AIDS. While they sought to educate, these media campaigns contributed to an atmosphere of fear and fatalism around HIV/AIDS.

Scholars working in South Africa have suggested that these early messages, emphasizing the lack of a cure for AIDS and the fatality of the diagnosis, articulated with religious and popular discourses to contribute to the construction of persons living with HIV/AIDS as being "dead before dying," leading to denial and silence.[21] For most of the 1990s, this silencing fear was not balanced by any apparent benefits to discussing AIDS. Not only was there no treatment for AIDS, there was no rapid HIV test. HIV was a clinical diagnosis, and people suspected of having AIDS were sent home in order to free up scarce hospital resources for patients with treatable illnesses. Doctors and other health workers often did not disclose the HIV diagnosis for a variety of reasons, from a reluctance to demoralize someone by giving them what amounted to a death sentence to a fear of triggering a last chance sexual rampage.[22]

In the mid-2000s, few Mozambicans living with HIV/AIDS were disclosing their status to others. On World AIDS Day in 2005, an expatriate organizer of an educational event complained that despite the growing cohort of people taking ARVs, she struggled to find a single person living with HIV/AIDS in Chimoio willing to publicly state their status and their experience seeking treatment for a public "breaking the silence" education event. Ultimately, it was mostly members of a youth AIDS education troupe who had to "break the silence" using fictitious names and experiences. The one speaker who did disclose his own HIV-positive identity covered his face while on stage. After the performance, rather than celebrate his disclosure, many in the large audience of several hundred Mozambicans questioned his motives, wondering why he covered his face and why such clearly fictitious accounts were presented to an audience full of people living with HIV/AIDS.

Silence surrounding a diagnosis was not necessarily related to apathy, denial, or ignorance. People were reluctant to "come out" as HIV positive for several reasons. Joaquim previously explained the widespread fear that being HIV positive made a person vulnerable to witchcraft. Another was a fear of abandonment. Tomas, an HIV activist I knew and one of the earliest recipients of ARVs through the NHS in Chimoio, was thrown out of his mother's house by his siblings after he talked of being HIV positive on national television in 2004. On a less public scale, an activist I knew was abandoned by her partner when she developed a cough three months after she tested positive and he tested negative. Such stories emphasizing the dangers of visibility for people with HIV circulated commonly in central Mozambique.

A reluctance to publicly break the silence also spoke to an ambivalence regarding the dynamics of the AIDS economy. Self-promotion was viewed with suspicion. Why would someone render themselves vulnerable in this way if they were not gaining from it? Indeed, people often were paid to break the silence.[23] In the speculation and hustle of the AIDS economy and the perception of both great opportunity and investment alongside exclusion and unrelenting hunger, many wondered whose interests were truly being served. Were the interventions there to care for the sick or to enrich the powerful at the expense of the sick? Such skepticism was commonly expressed in the idiom of witchcraft. Witchcraft accusations have long been tied to unnatural accumulation of wealth and power.[24] Witchcraft discourse in contemporary Africa has been mobilized to make sense of increasing social and economic disparities produced by neoliberal policies and to problematize the ideal of the independent individual that underlies neoliberal ideology.[25] Rather than being anachronistic, witchcraft remains a salient way to discuss "the tensions between individual agency and accumulation on the one hand and social obligations to kinship and collectivity on the other."[26]

The fear-based messages of "AIDS Kills" were countered by an empowerment approach that placed the self-reflexive individual at the center of HIV/AIDS policy and trained and "capacitated" that actor to deal responsibly with the risks associated with HIV infection.[27] The ambivalence about going public with one's diagnosis was related to long-standing cultural notions of vulnerability and witchcraft as well as suspicions regarding AIDS interventions themselves and their relationship to forces of immoral accumulation. Administrators of AIDS interventions, however, much like the organizer of the World AIDS Day "break the silence" event, understood this ambivalence as resulting from fear and ignorance. She was frustrated by what she understood as the persistence of apathy despite the arrival of ARVs and the "empowerment" agenda.

EMPOWERING AIDS ACTIVISM: *VIDA POSITIVA*

Since the lack of visibility of the epidemic was understood to be the principal barrier to combating the disease by international AIDS organizations, an approach was developed to explicitly counter this perceived denial and fatalism.[28] Inspired by the success of activists in the global north, particularly in the gay community, this approach positioned people with HIV/AIDS as central to fighting the pandemic by empowering them to "come out" and "give a face" to the disease.[29] In the global north, activism by people living with HIV/AIDS helped to reorient public health approaches to the epidemic from a narrow, biomedical focus on diagnosis and control to one of inclusion and empowerment.[30] Since HIV tended to affect already marginalized groups who were subject to discrimination, it carried considerable stigma wherever it appeared.[31]

AIDS activists in gay communities in the global north organized successful community-based prevention campaigns, such as posting explicit advice in bathhouses and providing care and support in the homes of sufferers, outside of biomedical institutions. Activists also lobbied the pharmaceutical industry, pressured regulatory authorities to fast-track drug licensing, and mobilized patients to participate in clinical trials.[32] The active involvement of people living with HIV was instrumental to these results. International organizations drew inspiration and personnel from these networks in the 1990s, bringing their experiences of community organization and patient empowerment to the global fight against HIV/AIDS. The notion that people with HIV/AIDS were positioned to be partners and leaders in the effort to address the epidemic became official policy at the 1994 Paris World AIDS Summit with the ratification of the Greater Involvement of People Living with AIDS (GIPA) initiative. GIPA was a mobilizing and organizing principle that recognized that the contribution of people living with HIV/AIDS was central to ethical and effective national responses to the disease.[33]

The empowerment approach was epitomized by *Vida Positiva*, which I was introduced to by Elena, an earnest and disciplined young AIDS activist with a quiet confidence whom I met in 2003, before ARVs were widely available. As she lamented their absence, I asked her what helped her survive. She showed me a pocket-sized *Vida Positiva* booklet. *Vida Positiva* was an education program on how to "live positively" through physical, emotional, spiritual, and nutritional techniques that countered the fatalism of "AIDS Kills." Living positively emerged in Uganda as early as 1987 and spread from there to elsewhere on the continent.[34] Adapted from the "positive health" program developed by psychoneuroimmunologist Neil Orr and twenty-year HIV survivor and activist David Patient in South Africa, *Vida Positiva* is rooted in an American tradition linking positive thought to health. The New Thought movements that date to nineteenth-century Christian Science emerged as scientifically informed Christian critiques that challenged mainstream religious and medical authority in the early twentieth century. Following in a long history of Christian belief in the healing power of faith, New Thought was an explicitly spiritual and Christian movement. "Positive thinking" would become secularized, psychologized, and medicalized during the twentieth century, emphasizing the healing power of an individual's faith in one's own self.[35] Many Mozambicans respiritualized *Vida Positiva*, which provided a discourse of hope and a set of self-care practices for people "*infected* and *affected* by HIV" (emphasis in original).[36] Those who could not access ARVs were urged to adopt the precepts of *Vida Positiva* in order to "live longer and more productive lives."[37] The *Vida Positiva* language was taken up and used by clinicians, caregivers, and people living with HIV/AIDS.

Launched in the early 2000s, *Vida Positiva* was disseminated through workshops, *palestras*, and a pocket-sized booklet distributed through clinics and NGOs (see figure 9). The pocket guide, which reached its third edition during my research, was divided into four parts:

The first part was an introduction containing brief biographies of two long-term survivors of HIV from before the advent of ARV treatment as well as basic biomedical information regarding HIV and AIDS, modes of transmission, and methods of prevention. Prominent in the introduction was "the recipe for survival: healthy body + healthy mind + healthy soul = long life." The reader was encouraged to ask the question "why live?" of him or herself.

The second section, "A Healthy Body: Diet, Exercise, and a Few Home Remedies," focused on health and nutrition, as well as techniques for water purification, personal hygiene, and menu planning, using materials that were theoretically available to the average Mozambican.

The third section was "A Healthy Mind: How to Effectively Deal with Stress and Emotions" and discussed hormones, the nervous

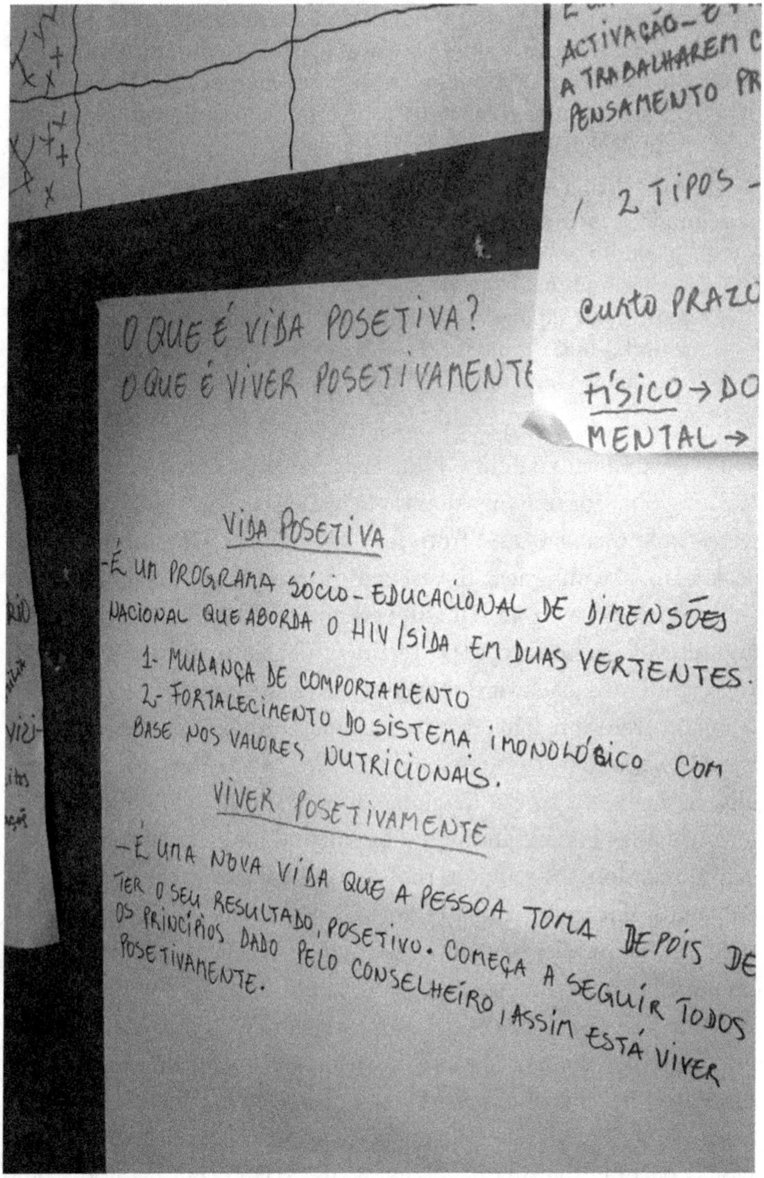

Figure 9. Precepts of *Vida Positiva* handwritten on posters at a *Vida Positiva* workshop.

system, shock, and how emotions affect health. It urged the reader to consider the future and to make at least three emotional objectives to aspire to. This section ended by encouraging HIV positive individuals to "talk to the virus"; "breathe"; and seek help, emotional or physical, when necessary.

The last section was entitled "Healthy Soul: Treating the Spirit," and reminded readers that they always have the liberty to choose the role of victim or to explore other options, that they should be grateful for life, and that love and prayer can be healing: "Our biggest strength is our capacity to choose—the freedom of choice. It is a gift from God. What should we do with our life? Feel like victims? Or believe that we have options?"[38]

Predicated on visibility, *Vida Positiva* provided a language for "coming out," for moving from the darkness to the light, from ignorance to knowledge, and from fear to hope. As HIV interventions scaled up, a willingness to test and pursue biomedical treatment was associated with an enlightened and civilized modernity, while an ambivalence toward AIDS testing and treatment was associated with ignorance, backwardness, and being stuck in African superstition and tradition. This duality was instantiated and reinforced in the AIDS economy through the discourse of *Vida Positiva*. Additionally, in a context where religion, Christianity in particular, plays a strong role in understandings of health and illness, temporality, and self-perception, the religious roots of positive living were exhumed. I frequently encountered the *Vida Positiva* booklets that were distributed by community organizations and in clinics in people's homes and association meetings.

Vida Positiva appealed to Mozambicans who strove to educate and improve themselves and to get ahead, who self-consciously embraced notions of modernity and progress. The language of *Vida Positiva*, oriented toward self-care, self-esteem, and the future, would become the lingua franca of the AIDS economy and would gain traction in a new set of interventions being scaled up in Mozambique in the early 2000s: community home-based care (CHBC), an approach training community volunteers in basic palliative care measures for the many people with HIV/AIDS who were being sent home from hospitals; associations of people living with HIV/AIDS, as sites of support and advocacy for people living with HIV/AIDS who may not have anywhere to turn; rapid testing associated with pre-and post-test counseling; and clinical services for addressing AIDS-related opportunistic infections. All of these approaches emphasized individual attitudes, behaviors, and choices.

EARLY AIDS ORGANIZATIONS: "FOOD IS MOTIVATION"

The first AIDS organizations in Mozambique were established in the 1990s in partnership with international organizations. Day Hospitals were established in 1996 in Maputo and in 1997 in Chimoio. CHBC organizations and associations of people living with HIV/AIDS also were created in the mid-1990s. Associations of people living with HIV/AIDS were founded in the spirit of the 1994 GIPA initiative, with the explicit purpose of fostering community-based networks of solidarity and support. These three organizations worked in concert. CHBC volunteers were the vanguard of an AIDS-focused response that tried to buttress the overwhelmed and underresourced NHS by caring for people in their homes rather than having them be admitted to hospitals. Nurses were involved in the first such effort to emerge in Maputo, but Chimoio's largest CHBC group was a faith-based community organization. The establishment of Day Hospitals addressed some of the burden of care for AIDS and provided specialty services, such as antibiotic prophylaxis for opportunistic infections and counseling. Associations often grew out of support groups that met in the Day Hospitals. An NGO coordinator in Maputo who helped organize an early association frankly described the stakes of membership: "They don't have a place to speak about their experiences. The messages have been 'AIDS Kills.' People felt outside of society . . .

[but] the first question is always, 'What are we going to eat?'" It was material support most members were primarily interested in, not the emotional and psychological support usually associated with support groups in North American contexts.

Solidarity and mutual support were often built on obtaining the necessities of living. Elena, who had introduced me to *Vida Positiva*, described the work and the situation of people living with HIV/AIDS in Chimoio:

> We are losing the sick (*estamos a perder doente*). If there was an organization to help with antiretrovirals. . . . They [antiretrovirals] are in the country, but they are expensive. Food, a few sick people receive from the World Food Program, but most of the members of the association don't have enough to eat. Transportation is an issue, supporting medications. Night and day, we think, how, how, how.

A founding member of one of Chimoio's early associations of people living with HIV/AIDS, Esperança [Hope], recalled shared food and medicine as a basis of emotional support:

> We'd get together like family and try to discuss some of our thoughts. We hugged, laughed, cried. We went to people's houses and invited them to join us, though all we really had to offer was compassion. We ate our African potato, tried to manage an egg every day.[39] We'd cook together and visit some of our neighbors who weren't well enough to join us.

The NGO coordinator explained, "Food is motivation." The primary concern of these associations was often basic survival.

As the numbers of people testing positive increased and the Day Hospital served more people, new associations were formed by entrepreneurial AIDS patients and organizations. This was not, strictly speaking, the organic emergence of mutual aid organizations at a grassroots level, but rather an entrepreneurialism driven by the resources that were available for associations in an emerging AIDS economy. Associations provided people living with HIV/AIDS with

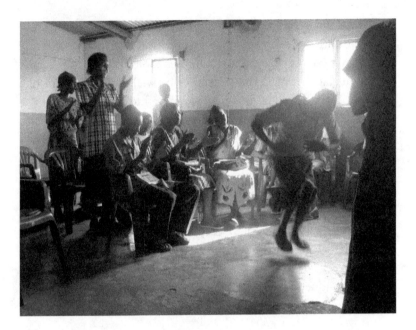

Figure 10. Association member expressing gratitude to other members through dance.

a peer group, solidarity, and friendship (see Figure 10), as well as counseling and education. Workshops trained members to work as neighborhood activists and conduct outreach, in the form of giving *palestras* about HIV at schools and workplaces and through counseling and care, both within the space of the association and through visits to the homes of ill kin and neighbors. Associations also sought to generate income by selling used clothes, dried bananas, and charcoal. One association arranged to grow vegetables to sell in the market. Another made and distributed their own herbal-based medicines to members of the association.

The weekly meetings and activities of associations fostered a community of fellow-sufferers who could counsel each other and benefit from workshops and trainings. In recalling his own experience living with HIV/AIDS, Diogo felt that it was not the disease itself that killed, but the isolation that often resulted from the disease, being left alone with one's thoughts: "Many die from rage, not the disease. Rage at not having anyone that consoles them. When I was alone, I thought many things, that I used to be well, and now I am like this, and I will die like this. I have no more life like this. It is those thoughts that kill." In the weekly meetings, seminars, and conversations in Chimoio's associations, the usual rules regarding talk about AIDS—silence, confidentiality, and euphemism—were inverted. Members freely spoke of their own and others' HIV status. In a context where people relied on social networks for survival, "psycho-social" support and material support were not easily separated. Suraia once asked me about employment opportunities, adding "that's why we go to the associations." The education and socialization she received at the association did finally lead to a contract with an NGO conducting HIV/AIDS education and outreach programs.

AIDS ENTREPRENEURIALISM

Dramatic increases in funding in the early 2000s made HIV/AIDS more visible in central Mozambique in multiple ways: through viral assays, population-level statistics, public performances of "breaking the silence," and T-shirts with printed slogans that reminded people "AIDS affects us all" (see Figure 11). Chimoio's city center was decorated with red AIDS ribbons that were painted on lampposts and walls by a youth group on a traveling national HIV education campaign in 2002. Radio spots advertised testing and treatment services. Educational songs recorded by a local NGO-supported group played on the community radio station and could be heard resounding throughout neighborhoods.

With the emphasis on participation and local partnership, the AIDS treatment scale-up unleashed a burst of AIDS entrepreneurialism. In his comprehensive account of the early response to AIDS in Mozambique, Mozambican anthropologist Cristiano Matsinhe

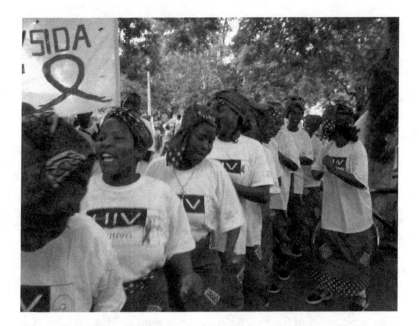

Figure 11. World AIDS Day Rally, Mozambique.

notes that hundreds of AIDS organizations of various sizes emerged across the country in the early 2000s, some seemingly created to expressly respond to funding requirements to partner with local organizations and to capture funds specifically targeting certain concerns or segments of the population. The result was organizations with awkward, formulaic names such as Association of Young Widows and Association of Single Fathers, with often just three members who fulfilled the official roles of president, vice president, and secretary or activist.[40] The National Council for the Fight Against AIDS found that there were few mechanisms to verify what activities specific organizations actually carried out and concluded that much of the information they provided was fabricated.[41]

Eusebio, a charismatic association member with a broad smile and confident swagger, seemed to embody the entrepreneurial spirit when he declared to me in 2005, "I am my own best resource!" He explained that the HIV positive status was gaining value, and with it, he was in demand with local NGOs. His organization was able to apply for grants and contracts: "The more people there are here with HIV, the more food we will get!" I was approached on multiple occasions, by strangers on the street as well as acquaintances and friends and family of acquaintances, with proposals for AIDS organizations that perhaps I would like to support or partner with. There was an urgency to this hustle, driven no doubt by poverty and desperation, but also the sense that one needed to get involved before the speculative AIDS scale-up bubble burst.

Eusebio's exuberant self-promotion seemed to evoke the spirit of the neoliberal figure of *homo economicus* that Michel Foucault referred to as an "entrepreneur of himself, being for himself his own capital, being for himself his own producer, being for himself the source of [his own] earnings."[42] Eusebio positioned himself as an AIDS entrepreneur, converting his diagnosis into a form of capital. The rapid influx of funding for AIDS treatment and the proliferation of organizations and interventions contributed to the emergence of an AIDS economy. Within this economy, HIV had a value that could be mobilized as a form of capital to be invested and to produce health and an income or wage, if not in cash then in the form of medical treatment, food, employment opportunities, and access to an exclusive network of organizations and fellow entrepreneurs. This was a competitive economy, however, as benefits were increasingly scarce as the numbers getting tested and treatment grew.

The arrival of treatment interventions, administered through government health clinics and NGOs, changed the "economic and the moral value of HIV."[43] They placed value on certain technologies and objects (HIV test results, antiretroviral medication, etc.), behaviors (taking the HIV test, "adhering" to ARVs, "breaking the silence," using a condom, practicing abstinence, etc.), and ways of "living positively" (planning for the future, abstinence from sex or using condoms, not taking herbal medications from *n'angas*, taking ARVs daily, eating a balanced diet, not smoking or drinking alcohol, etc.). Individuals who were able to adopt these behaviors and adapt to these norms and values gained access to the benefits of the AIDS economy.

AIDS treatment interventions offered a new way forward in a context of multiple competing sets of norms and values, in which survival was at stake. As treatment and support programs expanded, however, the number of those eligible for benefits far outnumbered their availability, and the scope of care provided increasingly narrowed. Accessing the scarce commodity of ARVs proved to require more than a positive test. People who were taking ARVs were grateful for the life their medication granted them. Yet the persistent hunger they felt, and the awareness of AIDS entrepreneurialism and the sense that, as Macamo wrote in a newspaper editorial, "there are those that live with AIDS and those that live off of AIDS," fostered an ambivalence among those struggling to survive on ARVs, a frustration that others were profiting from their suffering.[44] As AIDS and AIDS interventions became more visible in the early years of the twenty-first century, for many that visibility stood as a reminder of growing inequality and exclusion.

Many Mozambicans, even the HIV positive, cynically called the entire AIDS effort a business.[45] These comments are echoed in accounts of the AIDS pandemic elsewhere in Africa. In Uganda, "Fat AIDS afflicts doctors, bureaucrats, and foreign-aid consultants with enormous grants and salaries. Fat AIDS had become so common ... that if you said you were working on HIV, people thought you were a thief."[46] In Tanzania, AIDS was referred to as "The Acquired Income Deficiency Syndrome" and in Nigeria, AIDS was viewed by many as a boondoggle for government and NGOs.[47]

Conspiracy theories and suspicions swirled in the AIDS economy. There were rumors that some prominent association leaders were actually not HIV positive at all, but rather posing as positive in order to receive benefits. Indeed, one locally prominent association leader and HIV testing counselor was discredited and denounced when he was found to be HIV negative. I was told by activists who worked in the Day Hospital that another association leader was also HIV negative but pretended to be positive. Another association member disclosed to me that indeed she was not positive. She had been involved in the association from its founding and was allowed to remain in the group because she had some expertise in health care. She was assumed to be HIV positive by most association members, but the association head knew that she was not.

Stela, a young woman who had been recruited from an association of people living with HIV/AIDS to work in the Day Hospital, asked me:

> Is it true there is a secret about HIV? That they have the cure but don't let us have it because all these people would lose their jobs? I have heard that someone there made HIV just to then create all this work. If it were cured, what would all these groups [international NGOs] here do then?

This theory, that HIV had been invented "there," somewhere outside of Africa, in order to enrich international organizations, applies the observation that the AIDS economy seemed to enrich some while impoverishing others on a geopolitical scale. "You say you do not know of a cure, but I suspect they have one," Diogo, another association member recruited to work in the Day Hospital, added. He brought up his suspicions as well:

> Globalization works something like this. As population density increases, there is more hunger. Now, when population density decreases, there is less hunger. And then, this thing [HIV] appears. . . . This is a way of reducing [the population], until it reaches a certain number. We are dying! . . . This is another story, one that is not being told.

A darker narrative than Stela's, Diogo's story linked the development narratives of overpopulation, hunger, and AIDS in a nightmarish scenario meant to depopulate Africa that he termed "globalization." These rumors, that HIV was unleashed as a means of generating economic opportunities for foreign concerns, resonated with the

insecurities and fears of a chronically underemployed and malnourished populace in the midst of neoliberal reforms and an entrenched
local development economy, as well as with the long history of
extractive foreign intervention in central Mozambique.

These fears and anxieties speak to the kinds of unequal social
relations and hierarchies AIDS treatment interventions were contributing to. James Pfeiffer has described how, in keeping with the
neoliberal emphasis on privatization, international aid is channeled through NGOs and their expatriate technical experts. In Chimoio, this has resulted in growing local social inequalities as health
workers are hired away from the NHS by NGOs, and a class of local
and expatriate development elites has emerged.[48] In *The Republic
of Therapy: Triage and Sovereignty in West Africa's Time of AIDS*,
Nguyen argues that the emergence of AIDS treatment programs
contributed to a form of "therapeutic citizenship," in which having
HIV/AIDS "may be the only way to get access to forms of material security one usually associates with citizenship."[49] He asked
whether this would lead to increased competition and inequality,
or whether it may contain the seeds of new forms of belonging.[50]
I argue the embodied critiques and the suspicions of witchcraft and
even genocide shared by my interlocutors point to the meager benefit and divisive potential of therapeutic citizenship and the ways
this global health intervention inadvertently fostered exclusion
and discord. This therapeutic citizenship represents an entrenchment of neoliberalism, in which citizenship rights are devalued and
deferred in favor of market "governance." Rather than citizenship,
entrepreneurialism of the self is a more apt term, a process in which
the symbolic capital of the HIV diagnosis is exploited and used to
access scarce commodities. But simply having the diagnosis does
not grant access to benefits. Rather, it grants a person the possibility
of competing in the market of benefits.

Commenting on the inability of African governments to control
macroeconomic processes or to improve the daily living conditions
of the people, due in large part to structural adjustment measures

that undercut both sovereignty and resources, anthropologist James Ferguson notes that Africans increasingly "seek to find expressions of collective solidarity, social order, and moral beneficence outside of the state altogether," in local kin-based social systems, in ethnic separatism, in religiously inspired social movements, in millenarian cults, and in other movements aimed at "cleansing the world of its only too evident corruption and evil."[51]

SUBSISTENCE AS A MORAL CLAIM

Rita and Joaquim criticized the dynamics of the AIDS economy, lamenting the growing disparity between the powerful and those the powerful are supposed to serve:

> Things come from other countries, and they [the powerful and well-connected] take them. The money arrives, but it's not distributed, we don't receive anything. Even within the association, money comes, plans are discussed, but we receive nothing. Things come from other countries for us, and they are eaten before we get them, that is a great sin!

Rita accurately identified the site of the power, resources, and influence in global health as coming from the outside. She asked me to appeal directly to foreign donors rather than what she perceived to be an impotent and corrupt set of organizations, state and NGOs alike:

> Look, we are asking the whites, you can tell them, that when they bring things, they should bring them to us directly! Not give it to someone black like us. We won't be given anything! Things come; it's just they don't get to us. . . . Look at our house. Is this a house? When it rains, it rains inside and out. But people are getting rich, building houses with donor money.

This statement reflected Rita's perception that the resources of the AIDS economy were being captured by NGO administrators and other local officials. She pleaded with me, as a white representative of global health and development, for a direct connection to a powerful (white) patron. Her reference to race starkly underlined a continuity between colonial rule and the contemporary humanitarian enterprise. Rita made explicit what is often an "unacknowledged and unconscious assumption of white superiority and expertise within development as part of the wider, global distribution of racialized power."[52] The colonial distinctions of white versus nonwhite, civilized versus uncivilized have continued salience in the AIDS economy through the construction of whiteness and the West as symbols of authority, expertise, and knowledge. Even after the formal end of colonialism, the power imbalance was maintained thanks to the damaging effects of structural adjustment, which preserved the colonial economy of extraction and gave foreign powers more legitimacy and authority than citizens' own governments. Rita's view emerged out of the visible reality that the most vibrant economic growth seemed to be occurring in the humanitarian industry, specifically in relation to AIDS interventions, and an awareness that though HIV/ AIDS was a national and international priority, the material benefits that were desired proved to be elusive. Rita's comment also referred to fears that the unequal accumulation they witnessed was linked to the shadow economy of witchcraft and immoral traffic.

Joaquim cautioned: "If you see an African who is very rich, it's witchcraft from powerful herbal magic (*botânica*), drugs (*droga*)." This referred to a medicine that could turn people into zombies, whose labor could then be exploited without that person's knowledge or memory, and was often seen as the basis of large fortunes of wealth.[53] This was a critique of leaders who were enriching themselves at the expense of those they were meant to serve and was leveled at the then president Armando Guebuza, as well as at local association leaders. Knowing that being HIV positive made them all the more vulnerable to this treatment, they feared association leaders were scheming to exploit the labor of their members and were thus profiting from illness. That the ostensibly supportive space of the association could be used for the exploitation of the vulnerable bodies of its members underlines the profound ambivalence and sense of marginalization and abandonment that Rita and Joaquim themselves felt in relation to the AIDS economy. At the same time that they began ARVs, they sought solace and healing in the collective solidarity of their spiritual community and church that critiqued the corruption they saw as so pervasive in the world. Perhaps it was not a coincidence that Rita, with her lifetime spirit possession, also took their chronic illness seriously and encouraged her husband to do the same.

Joaquim remarked on the atmosphere of competition among people living with HIV/AIDS not only in association, but within households as well when he discussed their disappointment that only one of them could receive food allotments even though both were taking ARVs:

> Here we are, positivized. But this life is taxing! What really taxes us the most, is food. . . . [W]e don't have any. The association will only help one person, and each eats at the expense of the other. . . . [T]hat person is eating the blood of the other. If both of us in this house had enough, for two positivized people, then we could say things were a little normal.

Joaquim referred to himself and his wife as "positivized," embracing the HIV positive identity and acknowledging the transformation in subjectivity that they and others who lived positively underwent. He emphasized the contradiction that two positive individuals who belonged to an association, were adhering to their medications, and were doing all they could to be living positively, were still struggling because of their hunger. When I asked them if the allotment was not sufficient for two people, Rita responded, "But are we just two people? Do we not have family?" Whenever Joaquim and Rita brought the food they received from their association home, they were inundated with inquisitive kin, and they redistributed much of their grain among them. Even though the food was meant to serve as a part of Rita's medical treatment, and she was expressly told not to share it, keeping it to herself would have been a violation of the local moral economy and risked inviting either accusations of witchcraft or jealous attack.

This was what Joaquim referred to when he noted "each eats at the expense of the other." In order for one to eat, another goes hungry. By using the imagery of cannibalism, "eating the blood of the other," Joaquim evoked the zero-sum logic of the witchcraft economy, an economy of scarcity and illicit accumulation whose mechanisms are concealed. Antisocial witches consume human flesh, and Joaquim's somewhat ambiguous metaphor intimated that the inadequate distribution of food was sewing discord. Someone was eating the food meant for them, in effect eating their blood. Another interpretation could be that their own desperation might lead to one member of the couple turning on the other. While they shared their own food, they noted that this spirit of sharing and redistribution did not exist in the association and the AIDS economy more broadly. They experienced this as an abandonment and a violation of the relational moral economy of care, in which those who are better off must share a portion of their bounty with others.

Anthropologist Didier Fassin writes regarding subsistence as a moral claim: "A sense of injustice emerges as a result of the implicit agreement about the scope of tolerable exploitation being broken."[54] Fassin notes that James Scott, in his landmark work *The Moral Economy of the Peasant*, characterizes "the subsistence ethics" of peasants as organized around not the maximization of profit, as a liberal economist might presume of market actors, but around the minimization of risk because of the persistent scarcity of food. Fassin positions this "desire for security" as the foundation of "moral rights," including a "right to subsistence," in order to argue that "the nonobservance of these concrete principles in the past by the colonizer, and today by the state, international bodies, or NGOs, cause resentment and resistance, not only because needs were unmet but because rights were violated.'"[55] It is the violation of this right to subsistence that alarmed many Mozambicans struggling to survive on AIDS treatment, and that underlies the outrage expressed by the phrase "All I eat is ARVs."

When I first met Joaquim and Rita in 2005, they each appeared gaunt and weathered. They had sold most of their possessions in their struggles to survive their illnesses, and on my early visits to their home we sat together on a chunk of styrofoam and a plastic crate, as they did not own even one of the small wooden benches *bairro* families usually offered to guests. Five years later, things had changed for them. Both Rita and Joaquim had gained weight, and Rita's shiny cheeks fairly glowed. Yet this was not a case of the Lazarus effect, as there was more to their recovery than adherence to antiretroviral medication. Rita and her husband Joaquim belonged to an AIC, and the couple were regular attendees of the Saturday afternoon services. These were held outdoors in open fields on the outskirts of Chimoio; lasted several hours; and consisted of prayer, preaching, drumming, dancing, possession, trance, and healing. Pastors, *profetes*, and congregation members alike wore elaborate and colorful costumes that "both 'recall and scramble' a variety of Christian and medical referents."[56] Rita spent many of these ceremonies in the throes of possession, being administered to by healers as the service continued all around her. Rita explained that her relationship with the church was especially important in times of suffering and illness, when the pastor or members of the congregation would visit: "One person comes by, then another, to bring you a banana, bread, refreshment. Wash a dish or two. Or just to say hello and see that yes, you are still alive." This represents a much different ethos than the competition and scarcity of the AIDS economy.

Over the course of my fieldwork, Rita would go from being cared for by *profetes* in her church to becoming a *profete* herself. When I visited her in 2010, she was attending to the sick every day: "I once walked ill and I was told that I needed to start curing other people in order to get better myself, for my body to be well." It was through the harnessing of the spirit that possessed her, under the instruction of other healers, that she slowly began learning the practice. She did, however, distinguish between the sickness the spirit had caused and the HIV, noting that some things were better treated in the hospital. Visitors frequently called on her to minister to their various ailments. Rita's new vocation brought her not only increased visitors, but also status and material benefits, as those she cared for frequently brought her gifts of chickens, produce, and cash, at times amounting to 300–400 meticais per week (US$12–16). Joaquim also had managed to secure regular employment as a security guard for the warehouse of an Indian merchant, a job he found through contacts in his church.

Rita and Joaquim had found a way forward, one that involved ARVs, but which they did not wholly attribute to the AIDS economy or positive living. They drew on the multiple sources for support and therapy in the local relational economy of care. Indeed, they were disappointed by the opportunities they found within the AIDS economy, and they left their association. In 2010 they gleefully pointed to the wooden chairs they were able to offer me and other guests who visited, the mattress they now slept on, and their new zinc roof, laughing about the makeshift chairs we had sat on during the dark, uncertain days in which we met. Joaquim joked: "I was really preparing for my grave. I only had kept one pair of shoes and two sets of clothing." They were in a substantially better place than before. The case of Rita and Joaquim illustrates that despite the rigid precepts of *Vida Positiva* and the calls to abandon the backwards, ignorant ways of tradition, there were multiple paths forward through illness, suffering, and the AIDS economy.

3 Therapeutic Congregations

ASSOCIATIONS OF PEOPLE LIVING
WITH HIV/AIDS

The first AIDS support group in Africa, TASO (The AIDS Support Organization), began in Uganda in 1987 as an informal organization of friends.[1] It was founded by an HIV positive Ugandan expatriate after returning home who had learned about "positive living" approaches while in England.[2] The group adopted the slogan "Living Positively with AIDS" as a measure of defiance against the stigmatization and discrimination experienced by those living with HIV/AIDS. TASO quickly became an international role model. The founder of TASO and an activist from an NGO in Senegal created The African Network of AIDS Service Organizations in 1991, and in 1994 the Greater Involvement of People Living with AIDS (GIPA) initiative was ratified at the Paris World AIDS Summit, making associations of people living with HIV/AIDS part of a constellation of treatment techniques in the global scale-up. The first association of people living with HIV/AIDS was started in Mozambique soon afterward.

I met Elena—an activist member of Takashinga (We Were Brave)— in a cramped room in a house that a Christian AIDS organization rented for its office space. Then in her late twenties, Elena had been born in a village on the outskirts of Chimoio. Elena's father, a soldier, died when she was young. When her mother remarried, Elena was sent to live with her grandmother in Chimoio. She did not speak the local language, Chitewe, as she had learned her grandmother's tongue, Chigorongosa. Elena grew up in the Pentecostal church her grandmother belonged to, Apostolic Faith Mission's Church of the Apostles (Missão da Fé Apostólica, Igreja Fé dos Apóstolos).

Elena first began getting sick in 1999, with a stomachache, cough, and headache. Her mother had died of AIDS, and she recognized similarities between her own symptoms and those her mother experienced. When Elena's aunt heard about her "prolonged disease" (*doença prolongada*), she took Elena to get tested. Elena's aunt was also HIV positive and belonged to one of the first associations of people living with HIV/AIDS. Elena recalled her welcome from the head of the association, Isabela:

> We are sisters and brothers here. Your problem is the same that I have as well. Don't be afraid, we are family and we will help you. Whatever difficulty you may have, come and tell us.

Elena's own journey from uncertainty and repeated illness to recruitment by her aunt to get tested and join an association reflects some of the changing approaches to HIV that were emerging in the 1990s globally and in Mozambique. Originally, Elena was one of just six members of the Takashinga—she helped start its program of home visits, counseling, and outreach—but membership would grow. In 2004 there were only thirty-two members, but there were more than three hundred by the next year, reflecting the availability of ARVs and the increased investment in AIDS treatment interventions.

This chapter follows Elena's and others' experiences in the associations, where the terms of treatment were at times rehearsed, debated, resisted, embraced, ignored, or rejected. I term the collectivities that formed around AIDS and positive living "therapeutic congregations" because they combined practices and ideologies of healing churches and biomedicine.[3] This chapter also explores how testing positive and the practices of AIDS outreach and home visits were "evangelized" in the strong Pentecostal milieu of Chimoio's *bairros*, becoming narratives of rebirth and conversion. There was a tension in associations, and in the treatment programs generally, between notions of individual responsibility and moral worth and the collective solidarity and mutual support that these organizations were meant to foster. The second half of the chapter discusses the conflict that arose within associations over the scarcity of benefits and the exigencies of survival, revealing the impossible demands made by the precepts of positive living and individual responsibility in a context of austerity. This scarcity was due not to any absolute lack of resources—during the two decades following the civil war, Mozambique was one of the fastest-growing economies in Africa—but rather to the austerity measures imposed by structural adjustment. Structural adjustment funneled resources away from the public sector toward the private sector and NGOs while the majority of the population remained mired in poverty.[4]

CONVERSION: "I WAS DISCRIMINATED AGAINST AT HOME!"

Elena explained that there was still a lot of discrimination against people with HIV. She introduced me to a fellow association member, Florência, who was mentioned in the introduction. Florência had lived all her twenty-nine years between Chimoio and Catandica, the latter a town north of Chimoio near the Zimbabwe border. She married a soldier in 1995 and lived with him in Catandica, where she gave birth to a daughter. They separated in 1998, and she moved to Chimoio to resume her primary school studies. In Chimoio, however, she remarried and dropped out again during the last year of primary school. She had a son in 2002, but her husband fell ill during the pregnancy. She, her husband, and his family consulted a *n'anga*, who diagnosed the problem as being due to *vadzimu* on Florência's side, paternal ancestral spirits who had not been paid their proper respect. Despite repeated attempts to propitiate them, Florência and the newborn began having health problems as well. When her husband passed away a year after the child's birth, his family blamed Florência's accursed fate (*azar*), a term often used to refer to the misfortune that befell people who did not pay proper respect to ancestral spirits.[5]

Florência's in-laws passed their deceased son's very ill wife and child back to her mother so her own family could take care of her and give her a proper burial in her own family's house. They also feared that her presence would continue to bring the family misfortune, and they had already spent considerable resources on the multiple illnesses that had afflicted the household. By returning to Catandica with her mother, Florência would enter another complex set of familial tensions. Florência's father had passed away when she was young. Her mother had remarried and was living with her husband's family, to which Florência had no formal ties in the patrilineal kinship system. To make matters worse, Florência's health continued to worsen, and she was becoming an unwelcome burden on a family that did not consider her their own:

> They obligated me to sell off all my things—clothes, linens, dishes, everything—to pay for my food and care. But I don't know where everything went. They thought I was already dead. I could hear them fighting over what each would take.

Her mother's husband's family began to grow concerned about allowing Florência to die in their home because they would not be able to propitiate her ancestral spirits, which belonged to her father's lineage. Florência described the difficult situation her mother faced: "Her husband asked 'my dear, are you here for your husband or for your daughter who is sick and dying? She has done nothing but bring us problems.'" The expense of caring for her and the fear of ancestral recrimination again exposed Florência's precarious familial positioning. Her mother's in-laws demanded she be returned to her father's family, but Florência was not known to them, and they did not want to accept a sick and dying daughter simply to take on her burial costs.[6] Florência told me she understood her mother's position but nonetheless felt betrayed:

> I was discriminated against in my own home! My mother sent me away. She was tired of me. I would never be cured, my son was in the same situation, and my mother and her husband and his family could not take it, so they sent me away.

The family knew she was HIV positive, as she was tested again in the local hospital with her mother, and they thought Florência had brought her illness on herself. Caregiver fatigue was common in such settings, where chronic illness drained the already thin resources and energy of poor families. AIDS was described by one activist in Chimoio as "the guest that never leaves, that will consume all of our things and will finish us all." In the case of AIDS, families were faced with the choice of where to allocate scarce resources, a form of "lifeboat ethics" in which the "pragmatics of saving the savable" is evoked over more egalitarian principles.[7] Some families withdrew support from sick family members who were felt to be on the brink of death, in order to benefit the more productive members. AIDS activists frequently labeled such behavior *stigma* and *discrimination*, and Florência was using the language of these activists when she told me how her family had "discriminated" against her.

Florência was desperate. She turned to her neighborhood political leader, the *secretário do bairro*, who was able to give her a small, one-room shack on the edge of town. Home-based care volunteers from a local faith-based organization began visiting her, as did parishioners from a local Pentecostal church. They helped care for her, furnished her new home, and encouraged her to return to the Day Hospital, as treatment had recently become available: "I entered the church at the same time that I went back to the hospital and began treatment. The prayers really helped." She became one of the first members of a new association of people living with HIV/AIDS. She told me how she welcomed the solidarity and fellowship of her new church and her colleagues in the association:

> I had no help, no guidance, no support, nothing and no one. . . . When I began treatment, I was 24 kilos [54 pounds]. . . . When I went to the water pump, people fled from me. . . . I was so isolated. . . . I fetched water alone, cooked alone, took care of my son. . . . But I kept going to the association, kept taking my medicine, praying with my church, and I managed to overcome. . . . I began to recover, little by little. I gained weight and had a body again.

After she had regained her health and her life, Florência was able to reconcile and reshape her relationship with her family.

Elena explained that she often saw families rejecting their members who were HIV positive. It was this complicated phenomenon, with political and economic dimensions as well as notions of kinship obligation, that AIDS activists like Elena felt could be solved by better communication and education. She tried to educate families away from the belief that AIDS was caused by *uroi* or *azar*. Elena admonished families that just because something bad had happened to their loved one didn't mean that they themselves were bad. She compared it to malaria: getting bitten by a mosquito is bad, but that doesn't mean the person who got bitten is a bad person. The motto printed on one association T-shirt, *não é questão de azar; é prevenir*, is literally translated in English as "it is not a question of fate but prevention." However, the dilemmas posed by chronic illness in this context had less to do with ignorance and miscommunication and more to do with the exigencies of poverty, family history, conflicting etiologies of illness, and ties of obligation and familial belonging.

Along with two other association members who were fellow churchgoers, Florência broke the silence on World AIDS Day 2005 in Catandica, publicly speaking about her experiences being HIV positive and recovering with antiretroviral treatment. Her diagnosis granted her entry into a new social network. She framed her recovery as an explicit turn toward Christianity and biomedicine and away from "African tradition," a common discursive way of framing the "conversion" to positive living, echoing the Pentecostal practice of "breaking from the past."[8] She also used this language to disparage the way she was treated: "This is tradition you see? Tribal customs. African things." She evoked the tradition-modernity dualism that was heavily resonant with biomedical-evangelical parallels to emphasize that she was moving forward into modernity and health and leaving African tradition behind.

ACTIVISM, ARVS, AND EVANGELISM

The evangelical practices of Pentecostal churches and the educational practices of public health outreach came together in the home visits activists made. When Takashinga was still just a handful of people, Elena began accompanying CHBC volunteers on home visits. As Takashinga grew, Elena helped the association formalize its own home visit program. Elena's lived experience with HIV/AIDS and with testing and treatment in the Day Hospital made her a particularly effective counselor and a persuasive outreach worker. Elena was unmarried and had no children, though she cared for her younger siblings, who were considered "AIDS orphans." She was young and soft spoken, with a gentle demeanor. She joked that people often doubted whether she was truly HIV positive, laughing while she recounted the words of one incredulous man: "You are lying, fat and pretty like that, you can't be positive! You are just eating money." He suspected her of posing as HIV positive in order to "eat money"—to illegitimately access the benefits of the AIDS interventions. Elena began carrying proof of her positive test with her. On her visits, Elena explained: "I encourage patients to take the test. I serve as an example: 'I took this path—testing, treatment—and look at me, I'm normal.'" People often took time to agree to be tested, over several visits spaced days, weeks, or even months apart: "We get to know the person, we cultivate familiarity. After a while, we might mention AIDS. We speak directly about what the HIV test is and explain the advantages and disadvantages. We explain the difference between AIDS and HIV."

Association members chose different neighborhoods each week in which to visit existing members as well as nonmembers who were sick, to encourage them to be tested and consider joining the association. They also would visit members who had been absent for an extended period or who were ailing and in need of assistance with daily chores and tasks. A visit might simply consist of a prayer and encouragement. It could include organizing assistance with cooking, cleaning, a bicycle ride to the hospital, or filling a prescription. These visits were modeled on those conducted by neighborhood churches and were a way of demonstrating solidarity and lending support as well as recruiting new seroconverts to the association. Updates were then given to the rest of the association at meetings, along with requests for visits to individuals who would benefit. When there were donor funds available, those conducting the visits received stipends of 60 meticais (~US$2.50) per day of visits. Visits were often still conducted even when funds were not available. Each week's visits were scheduled during the meeting, and the weekly schedule was posted. Activists made a record of the visits, in order to provide documentation for reports to donors. An activist would often record basic information about each home that was visited: name, age, family members living in the home, whether the individual had been tested or not, and a brief synopsis of the situation encountered.

Elena began visiting Julia, who lived nearby, after Julia's husband became ill. Elena offered help with cooking and caring for the children. Julia recalled Elena subtly asked if she and her husband had been tested for HIV by using euphemisms for testing, such as "Do you know your state of health? Have you really explored every possibility?" Julia reflected:

> Elena converted me. She saved me. She never got tired of visiting me, even when I did not want to test. Finally, when I fell sick another time I went with her to get tested. I'm really grateful for her.

Julia explained this to me one day when I visited her in a densely populated neighborhood of Chimoio. We sat in her front yard in the shade of her thatched roof, leaning against the cool wall of her mud-and-wattle hut. She wore a pink T-shirt with the outline of a fish that said "Jesus" on it. A year and a half earlier, she had suffered a miscarriage; her husband had fallen ill around the same time. They consulted a *n'anga*, who diagnosed the problem as being due to *vadzimu*. "We spent thousands of meticais on treatments, but nothing helped. I did not realize at the time what a waste that was. The *n'anga* was telling us lies, it is just a business." Elena was sarcastically derisive as she agreed: "*N'angas* are expensive! They just want money. I prefer spending my money on clothes, food. Traditional healers say you are sick because of an evil spirit."

Stories of the trajectory from illness, isolation, ignorance, and vice to fellowship, enlightenment, and positive living through sero-conversion and religious conversion highlight the religious, Protestant roots of positive psychology in *Vida Positiva* that found fertile ground in the Pentecostal fervor of Chimoio's peri-urban milieu. The moral discipline of Pentecostal churches appealed to Julia in her own efforts to stay adherent to ARVs.

Gonçalo, whom I had met in 2004 and accompanied as he tested positive and joined an association, made the resonances explicit when he explained why he had joined a church, after he already had become an association leader:

> It is recommended to frequent church because it is based on mutual respect. When you go there, you forget about your vices. The church prohibits drinking and smoking, and you can't just wander any which way you want. That's why a person should enter a church, to correct these difficulties.

Many of the precepts for living positively were similar to the codes of personal ethics encouraged in Pentecostal churches. Gonçalo saw church membership as a way to reinforce good habits and behavior. He noted that his CD4 count increased after he joined the church, stopped drinking, and started going to sleep earlier.[9] He often compared the association to a church while speaking to members at meetings:

> The association is for living together, for you to come and de-stress yourself, to speak of the problems you confront at home, alone. Here we all have the same problem, and we can forget it for a while. . . . Through the association you have friends; you have family. It's the same thing as a church. You go to find family. Because in the suffering of one, others participate.

Elena's skill, commitment, and integrity earned her a reputation within Takashinga such that volunteers would consult her at home and, as treatment expanded, Day Hospital patients would do the same. On my visits to Elena, as we sat chatting in her *quintal*, patients, family members, and volunteers would drop in with questions or messages. Often they were Day Hospital patients who ran out of medications on the weekend. If she was taking the same line of medication, Elena would give them some of her own and ask them to return the medication after they got refills. If she was not taking the same line (there were only two lines), she would direct them to someone who was. At times she was called on in moments of crisis; she recounted the story of a man who breathlessly pulled up on a bicycle as she was preparing dinner late one afternoon, "*Dona* Elena, we need you, urgently!" She accompanied him to his house, where his wife lay inside, sweating profusely and with labored breathing. Along with a volunteer, they brought her outside to make her more comfortable and to figure out a way to get her to the hospital, but "we did not realize it was just to bid her farewell"; Elena described her breathing grow more ragged and irregular, until it stopped in the course of the next few minutes. She shook her head; "it was all too late." Elena reflected on the suffering she encountered: "Pain reminds us of Jesus. If everything was fine, happy, easy, we would forget God. This [pain] reminds us of God."

Elena often expressed frustration and anger over what she saw as treatment delays that could result in unnecessary deaths: "Those who know they are sick, that they may have AIDS, they don't want to go [get tested]. Even if they have the clear signs, they don't go. They say 'I know I may have AIDS, but I don't want to know.' They want to stay in the dark." She explained why she thought AIDS was feared and why few people willingly talked about it: "People think that they receive the result and life ends there. But they can have more life. It's a new life. Sometimes they will accept and change their vices. They can enter and change their behavior."

I would learn that this was a characteristic way of talking about AIDS in the associations. Prior to the availability of ARVs, AIDS was understood as a death sentence that placed people in a limbo of being "dead before dying," leading to fears of pollution and contamination that had less to do with notions of HIV transmission than with long-standing rituals and proscriptions around death.[10] Testing was associated with clarity and light. ARV treatment seemed to provide a way forward, to a new life after "death before dying." Activists like Elena saw themselves as spreading this good news, the gospel of treatment. The activists saw themselves as leading people out of "death before dying," away from isolation, ignorance, and darkness into fellowship, knowledge and light. They frequently described their own journeys in this manner. AIDS was also tainted with immorality. Despite the fact that HIV could be transmitted through nonsexual means, such as blood transfusions and contaminated needles, the underlying assumption was that to become HIV positive, someone must have done something wrong, and thus they were usually the target of judgment and blame.[11] Testing and joining the association offered a path to moral redemption. A refusal to get tested was associated with denial, fear, and ignorance.

HEALING BODIES AND SAVING SOULS

Biomedical and Pentecostal modes of self-care came together around positive living and taking ARVs, which a Day Hospital counselor referred to as "our daily bread." The language of counseling linked faith in clinical care to salvation, and traditional medicine to deception, exploitation, and ignorance. In Takashinga, not only did individuals frame their own experiences in this language, but many simultaneously drew on faith healing while adhering to biomedical treatment regimens.

In addition to accompanying Elena on some of her home visits, I met and accompanied Lucia, a *profete* who belonged to Takashinga and subsequently became the leader of an association in a small town in Manica Province. Her grandmother had been a *n'anga*, and Lucia had inherited her spiritual gift for healing (*dom*). "You may die, get sick, or go mad if you try and deny it," she explained. The turn to Pentecostalism was therefore less a true break with the past than a refiguring of her relationship with the past in order to strategically position herself in the present.[12] Lucia pursued mentorship from a *profete* in a Zionist church, rather than from a *n'anga*, to learn to master this *dom*. Getting trained as a *n'anga* would have been more time-consuming and expensive, and she felt she would have trouble getting married because men would fear the spirits who would have surrounded her. She explained that there was no problem in combining faith healing with biomedicine, partly because faith healing often did not involve the ingestion of medicines, unlike the herbal treatments of *n'angas*.

I accompanied Lucia when she visited another association member, Celeste, who was suffering from diarrhea and severe nausea through her initial weeks on ARVs. When we arrived at her house, along with three other activists from the association, Celeste was seated on *esteira* in her *quintal*, hunched over in discomfort. Lucia sat beside her and offered her hand, which Celeste grasped tightly. The activists all began to sing a popular gospel song in Chitewe,

"Taura ne mi Baba" (Speak to me, God) and clapping, and we all moved inside, where Lucia entered into a trance and then into a dialogue with the spirit contributing to Celeste's ailments. She dramatically recited a prayer and a blessing over a cup of water and a bit of salt, which she dispersed around Celeste's body and her hut. Pastors performed a similar ritual on home visits to congregation members. This had a protective purpose.[13] As Lucia explained, people who were already ill were easy targets for malevolent spirits. She frequently treated these problems in members of the association. Isabela, also a *profete* as well as the head of Takashinga, explained:

> When people are sick, they seek God. Here, where we create a place for the sick, we also need to consider this religious element. First, people come here looking for brothers and sisters, then to seek help. This is where they find God as well. We pray and explain the correct path to living positively.

She saw the religious component as an essential therapeutic aspect of what the association offered, which complemented the biomedical orientation.

I never got a sense that activists were overtly proselytizing for specific churches or denominations, though certainly people freely switched churches, and some people whom activists had helped did join their churches. Most were oriented to the pragmatics of healing and survival. Many association members I knew sought faith healing regularly, outside the association in their own churches. One day, while I was in the waiting area of the Day Hospital, Amílcar, an association member, surreptitiously lifted his shirt sleeve to show me the red string he wore, a protective measure used in AICs by people who were vulnerable to spiritual attack, such as children and ill individuals. The blending of spiritual healing with biomedicine that occurred in the associations follows a long history of missionary medicine in Africa, "healing bodies and saving souls."[14] In this case, it was not foreign missionaries proselytizing the natives to convert to Christianity, but rather local AIDS activists, empowered by

Vida Positiva, encouraging the ill to get tested and avail themselves of treatment. The presence of *profetes* in the associations and the deployment of Pentecostal healing practices on AIDS outreach visits reflected a pragmatic and eclectic therapeutic and spiritual approach common in Mozambique.

AIDS activists did bring an ideological fervor to denouncing *n'angas* and "African tradition," however. While *profetes* and spiritual healing were embraced within the associations, *n'angas* were not. Associations prepared their own herbal medications and mocked *n'angas* as dishonest charlatans and vestiges of an ignorant past. Consultations with *n'angas* and failure to promptly seek biomedical care were seen as signs of a pathological subjectivity marked by ignorance and individual failure. The path to ARVs and to living positively was seen to require a conversion to a more individualist, future-oriented, and cosmopolitan subjectivity. In associations, much as in the Day Hospital, the forward-looking, modern individuals who lived positively were contrasted with those oriented toward the past, who preferred healers to hospitals and whose ignorance and cultural practices were said to put them at risk of HIV. On this point, the framework of positive living within the associations was fairly rigid.

Gonçalo explained this framework to me:

> A positive life is a life in which a person leaves their old habits and passes into a new life. Life has to start over, practically from the start. You change your behavior, you have to abandon your vices and consider your future. I used to be out of control, didn't pay attention to how I ate. I used to drink a lot of beer, stayed up all night. I smoked. I didn't care about condoms. If you had a lot of partners, you have to just stay with one. You have to use a condom as your basic tool, and also not have sex frequently. You have to have a balanced diet. You can't be up all night. Also to not upset yourself too much, to not create stress, and to not visit the *n'anga*. When a person can live according to these rules, then a person is living positively, and he may live longer.

This list of behavioral proscriptions and prescriptions was often recited in rote fashion by people with AIDS who had been counseled in the clinic or in associations. There was a distinct moralizing tone in the language about vice, the value of monogamy, and avoiding the *n'anga*. This moralizing tapped into ideologies of civilization and moral purity accompanying Portuguese colonialism and the postcolonial state-building project in Mozambique, which also resonated strongly with contemporary Pentecostal church movements in Chimoio.[15] Metaphors of moving from the darkness into light were frequently used to describe the awakening that occurred following testing positive and joining the association. Testimonials and conversion were keys to the performance of positivity that demonstrated a moral rehabilitation and proper comportment.

AIDS TESTIMONIALS

In 2003 I spoke to Elena about her personal experiences living with HIV/AIDS. She told me that in addition to making visits, such as those helping Julia, and encouraging testing, she and other activists gave talks at schools and workplaces. These testimonials, based on *Vida Positiva*, were also delivered to associations throughout the central region. It was a national education and outreach program, taught in clinics and community organizations, to empower individuals with knowledge, techniques for self-care, and hope. These testimonials reinforce a kind of personal responsibility by suggesting, as the slogan on the cover of the second edition of the *Vida Positiva* booklet stated, "Yes I can! So can you" (*Sim, eu posso! Tu também*). The back of this booklet featured the accompanying slogan, "I take it on, and you?" (*Eu assumo, e tu?*). Both emphasize the neoliberal notions of self-responsibility, self-control, and self-determination and the idea that healthy living entails making the right choices and adopting the proper outlook.

Many in Chimoio infused the language with an evangelical fervor. This was dramatically illustrated to me in a spirited sermon that opened a *Vida Positiva* seminar with Takashinga that I attended in Chimoio in July 2004:

> The Prophet Ezekiel was sitting at home when God called him. He was taken to a valley full of dry bones. He looked around, shocked, and saw that these bones were the bones of people. The Lord said to Ezekiel, "Evangelize! Tell these dry bones to hear the word of God, and I will grant them new life!"

The speaker, Fernando, was an officer of Takashinga and a youth minister in his church. Fernando and Elena were both first involved in their churches before becoming HIV positive AIDS evangelists. Fernando addressed an audience of around twenty HIV positive individuals on the third day of a five-day seminar. Some had recently joined the association; others had been active for a few years. They sat on the concrete floor or in plastic chairs underneath a corrugated zinc canopy in the back yard of the offices of Mufudzi.

> So Ezekiel obeyed him: "You, dry bones, hear the word of God!" he said, and he heard a great noise. What was this great noise? The bones began to move, from the place they lay, to the place they belonged. The skull ran to the vertebrae, and then came the hips, shoulders, legs, arms, each bone in its place, and the bones became a valley filled with skeletons.

Fernando's reference to a valley of bones left behind by a great war may have resonated with his fellow Mozambicans who had lived through at least part of the fifteen-year civil war that ended in 1992 and preceded a decade of austerity and the rise of the HIV epidemic. He brought in the bodily imagery of flesh, bones, sinew, and blood, which spoke to the ravages of illness many in Takashinga were experiencing. But he also evoked the possibility for renewal, growth, and solidarity:

> "I evangelize! You dry bones, grow muscle, tendons, nerves, flesh, and blood!" The bones grew muscle, flesh, blood, and skin. And the Lord

sent a great wind, and the people began to breathe, and when they
saw they were alive again, they began to move, to play, to dance, and
to live.

Fernando wove the struggles those living with HIV faced in Chimoio
into a retelling of an Old Testament passage:

> We here today, are like these bones, we have come here looking for
> new life, for words that may feed and nourish us. But we must hear
> the Word, hear and understand what will be transmitted today. And
> then, we must animate those words, and pass them on to others like
> us, giving them new life as well.

He spoke for many of those present when he referenced a search
for new life, for knowledge, and for material sustenance: money
and food. At the time of this seminar, treatment had just become
available, and the majority of those present were not enrolled in
treatment.

> Many people don't understand: *Vida Positiva* is a new life. Many
> whisper, we want a coffin to hide in, we want money to live.... [I]t's
> a great struggle, people, a war.... I, who know my state of health, I
> will live. All of us here today, we know our state of health. We have
> come together so that we may live and to learn how to help ourselves,
> and to help each other.

Fernando's sermon seamlessly integrated Christian notions of the
Word and divine healing power with *Vida Positiva* and one's "state of
health" (*estado de saúde*), a euphemism for HIV serostatus, a clinical
test result. Fernando's sermon, however was less about individuals'
orientation to themselves and their illness and more about coming
together as one in the association to aid each other. In this way it was
not a typical *Vida Positiva* testimonial. Rather, it shows how associations built on locally meaningful experiences and priorities to foster
solidarity and support.

At another presentation in Chimoio's Takashinga, Bruno recounted
his personal story and experience with ARVs:

A normal person has a CD4 of 1000, 2000. It's a defense from disease, and when CD4 is finished, you are eaten. I reached this phase—I had to be transported from hospital to home, home to hospital. I had no hope that I'd live. I was looking for some way of explaining this, to explain why my life was leaving me. And where did I go? Of course, I went to those who told me it was a problem with my ancestors, with my house [n'angas]. But I did not improve. Now, when I went to the hospital, I tested positive for HIV. I had a CD4 analysis. I had 35. A nurse said, "sir, your life is at risk. Start taking this, and tell me how it is. I am at your disposal." So, on the 16th of August, 2004, I began taking antiretrovirals. I wouldn't be here today if I hadn't begun this treatment.

Bruno raised his bottle of ARVs, to applause and cheers (see figure 12). He smiled and dramatically added: "After six months, I went to get a follow-up count, and my CD4 had jumped to 197! My most recent count was 425 and I haven't had any problems with malaria, headaches, nothing!" The audience, around fifty men and women, burst into applause, energized by Bruno's charismatic presentation. Some eagerly offered their own success stories. Tomas, one of the first in Mozambique to embrace ARVs and "break the silence," called out from the audience: "I had a CD4 of 39 initially, and I am great now! I owe my life to the treatment and everything I've learned in the association!" Similarly enthusiastic testimonials ensued, following a familiar pattern that could be seen as a script within associations, of falling sick, searching in vain for answers, going to traditional healers but not improving, and finally taking the HIV test and starting ARVs. New members introduced themselves to associations using the same script, as did public presentations of "breaking the silence." These testimonials drew on the same narrative and performative repertoires I heard in local Pentecostal churches and that are common across Africa: public accounts of people overcoming hardships and fighting against the odds before finally moving out of darkness and achieving a transformation of the self.[16]

Testimonials, conversion stories, home visits, and hybrid healing practices all served to unite people in their experience of a rebirth

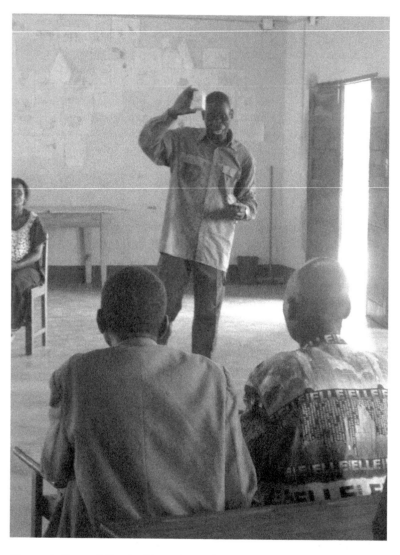

Figure 12. Bruno delivering his testimonial at an association meeting.

into positive living and their rejection of an ignorant past, symbolized by repeated trips to *n'angas*. By performing testimonials, people declared that they were forward-looking, modern individuals who were living positively and taking responsibility for themselves. The testimonials that were shared privately, by Elena, as well as publicly, by Bruno, reinforced that simply testing positively did not mean one was living positively. The testimonial was a public acceptance of "the truth" of the biomedical test and a rejection of the ignorance symbolized by the *n'anga* and "African tradition." It was also common to lament the poor treatment suffered at the hands of family members while one was in the worst stages of illness and to blame this on tradition or African culture, in distinction to the cosmopolitan modernity of the AIDS economy. Similarly, with the benefit of hindsight, association members frequently characterized the time and resources they had devoted to traditional therapies as a waste when they ultimately tested positive.

Born-again testimonials might include breaking with an ignorant past in which answers were sought from *n'angas* or signs of AIDS were not recognized. Or testimonials could include the rejection of an immoral past, of promiscuity and poor decisions. By emphasizing becoming born again as a complete break with the past, individuals born again as HIV positive distanced themselves from the immoral and ignorant past that led to their infection and emphasized individual responsibility for health and avoiding affliction. In this way relational etiologies of affliction as well as revolution-era Frelimo's calls for solidarity and individual sacrifice for collective benefit contrasted with the neoliberal stance of the contemporary government prioritizing individual responsibility and choice.[17] With the relational idiom of disease, responsibility for causing illness lies outside the person, with unseen others such as *uroi* or spirits, and the resolution frequently involves identifying the perpetrator. Anthropologist Susan Reynolds Whyte notes that unlike with suspicions of *uroi*, which posit intent, AIDS is not transmitted through malice, but rather through individual immorality, carelessness, and irresponsibility. She suggests that AIDS "is contributing to the emergence of a new idiom of action in relation to the uncertainty of misfortune: an idiom of individual responsibility for avoiding affliction."[18]

The assumptions of positive living oversimplified and misrepresented the predicaments individuals faced as they negotiated survival in the AIDS economy. In many ways, positive living made impossible demands on people and denied the complex realities of livelihood, sustenance, and reproduction. It did not sufficiently account for the risks of being seen as HIV positive in certain contexts. Nor did it account for the structural dynamics of the epidemic that rendered the poor and women more vulnerable. This oversimplification, which overemphasized the role of the individual and obscured the role of social and political relations in the epidemic, mirrors the simplistic message of the Lazarus effect.

When Oswaldo, a local activist, fell sick and tragically died within the span of a few months, people speculated about his unhealthy behaviors and immoral choices—smoking, drinking, unprotected sex—rather than lamenting the fact that there were not enough second line ARVs available for those in whom the first line failed, or that Oswaldo struggled to feed his family after losing his job in the Day Hospital just prior to falling sick. Oswaldo suffered due to an inadequate health and social infrastructure and lack of employment opportunities, both of which are connected to policy decisions made outside of Mozambique. Yet the emphasis on *Vida Positiva* and individual responsibility blamed him for his own demise.

"MY HEALTH HAS CHANGED BUT MY DIET HAS NOT"

During the discussion that followed Bruno's testimonial, Batista offered an alternative account: "My health has changed but my diet has not. There are fourteen people in my house who need to eat. I appreciate the food I receive, but there are days when I just don't eat." Batista received a monthly World Food Program (WFP) food supplement from the association, which in 2006 consisted of 36 kg of rice, 18 kg of corn-soy blend, 6 kg of beans, and 1.5 liters of oil. But it rarely lasted two weeks when distributed among kin. Suzana, an activist who worked in the Day Hospital, responded to him in the same manner she would have in the clinic:

> Sometimes we create laziness ourselves. You're sick, it's true, but the mouth doesn't close. Is this disease going to pass? No. So you better change your attitude and your thoughts. Thinking a lot, about your misfortune, is the worse disease you can have.

This response silenced Batista's talk of hunger. It directed attention to his attitude and thoughts rather than his, or his family's, empty bellies and the broader economic and structural forces implicated by their hunger. It was characteristic of how hospital providers individualized AIDS and pushed the responsibility for survival onto patients. This was how the doctrine of *Vida Positiva* created people who lived positively: people were told not to complain about what they needed. Those who lived positively did not ask for help but were resourceful and entrepreneurial.

While associations did offer food supplements and other material benefits, the scarcity of these benefits led to competition and strained their attempts to foster solidarity. Members tended to be poor and unemployed. Calls for solidarity that did not address their material needs rang hollow, particularly while associations were expanding within the burgeoning AIDS economy. In the early days of the associations, when membership was small and programs were just beginning, all regular members received food aid and participated in training. Associations grew to such a degree, however, that there were waiting lists for food aid and for entry into educational seminars and workshops. As the clinics and NGOs expanded their HIV programs, they recruited association members for long- and short-term work. These more substantial benefits were often

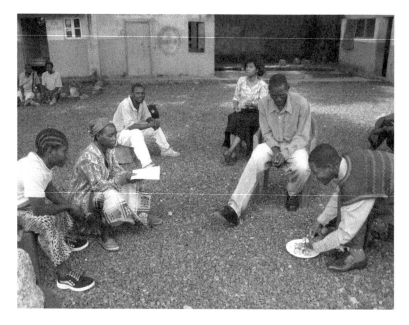

Figure 13. Association members sharing cucumber after a meeting.

distributed as rewards for loyalty and service. Occasionally, smaller benefits, such as T-shirts, pairs of shoes, *capulanas*, and association-made aloe vera balm, were also distributed. Those who were lucky enough to attend a multiday workshop or seminar often ate two loaves of bread as well as a lunch each day (see figure 13). Lucia once remarked to me, "We get fat during seminars!" Association meetings ended with the distribution of bread. This meal, literally breaking bread together, was a powerful symbol of solidarity and sociality. At one Takashinga meeting, however, the bread ran out before everyone had received a piece, and a chaotic free-for-all broke out as the empty-handed all made for the last remaining bag of bread. Even those who received food, however, might go hungry.

Many of those who had recovered their health with ARVs found themselves much worse off than they had been before falling ill, as many had sold all their assets to pay for treatments and had lost spouses and family members to the disease. Batista lived with three adults and ten children, six of whom were his deceased brother's, in his household. Batista usually ate the staple diet for the region: manioc or sweet potato for breakfast with some tea and a corn meal porridge (*sadza*) with a relish made with some leafy greens, often pumpkin, cowpea, or sweet potato leaves (*massemba*) later in the day. When funds were available, this was supplemented with legumes, groundnuts, or dried fish (*matembe*). *Matembe* was the main source of protein, but it was relatively expensive (~US$1/kg), and Batista could not tell me the last time they had eaten a chicken in his house. Occasionally during the dry season, his sons would trap field mice outside the city to supplement their diets and to sell in the market. His wife and sister worked in the *machamba* (small familial agricultural plot), twenty kilometers outside the city, but the fourth consecutive year of erratic rainfall yielded less than a two months' supply of grain from the *machamba*.

Batista had worked for TextÁfrica for eight years, until it closed in 2000. After he lost his job, he got by on short-term work opportunities as a welder until he fell sick. He was unable to work for nearly a year and sold some of his welding equipment, as well as his bicycle and radio, to pay for visits to various healers and clinics before he tested positive. He still occasionally found work welding, but he complained that he lacked his previous stamina, and his unpredictable health status could cost him workdays and make him a liability to rehire. He might earn 300 meticais (US$40) in a good month. The estimated cost per person, per day of basic nutritional requirements in urban Manica was estimated to be 9.6 meticais (~40 US cents).[19] For his family of fourteen, this would come out to just over 4,000 meticais per month, thirteen times what he typically earned. His wife and eldest two children also chipped in earnings, but the family's pooled monthly income rarely approached a thousand meticais.

Discontent about access to benefits was at the heart of an acrimonious split in Takashinga in 2005. At the time, Takashinga was the largest association in Chimoio, with close to four hundred official members. The group had a legacy of disappointing efforts to stimulate income-generating activities. An accountant hired to help Takashinga organize its finances told me this was due to poor management and communication. Within the association, the disappointment usually incited accusations of corruption and witchcraft. A disagreement in how food aid should be distributed led some members of Takashinga to break away and form their own association, Association of People Taking Antiretrovirals (Associação de Pessoas Tomando Medicação Antiretroviral; APToMA).[20] The group's focus on not just people living with HIV but also people taking ARVs was a savvy attempt to capitalize on the emphasis being placed on the treatment scale-up.

APToMA's main patron was a retired ministry of health employee who had emerged as a local AIDS entrepreneur. He had helped found a few successful AIDS organizations in Chimoio since the mid-1990s, and he took the fledgling organization under his wing. He built an oven for baking bread that association members then sold, splitting their earnings with him. They applied for and were awarded a "small grant" from PEPFAR totaling US$20,000, quite a boon for the sixty-odd members, and managed to fulfill the administrative requirements for accessing the funds despite having neither an office nor a computer nor a member who could type. APToMA received the grant in 2006 and used the funds to build a humble brick-and-mortar, two-room office in an expanding residential neighborhood on the outskirts of the city, to manage a *machamba* yielding produce for consumption and sale that included hiring laborers, and to purchase a mill for corn that they would charge local residents for grinding. All this was in addition to home-based care, home visits, education, and outreach. The group received US$16,000 from the original grant and was also awarded a renewal grant of US$14,000. Unlike Esperança and Takashinga, one of APToMA's strategies for ensuring that benefits could be distributed to all members was to make membership more exclusive and to restrict the number of members.

"WHAT ABOUT SEX?" LOVING WITH HIV/AIDS

The topic of sex and reproduction was another source of controversy in associations. After a meeting discussing sexually transmitted diseases that emphasized that ARVs would not prevent their transmission, Carmen, an irreverent association member in her late twenties with short hair and flashing eyes, expressed some confusion to the dozen members still gathered: "Some say that with ARVs we can live normally, and here we are talking about STDs, but what about sex?" She went on to say that she thought living positively meant no longer having sex at all. Her confusion was the result of conflicting messages about sex and fertility that were circulating. Clinic providers clearly stated that HIV positive people were never to have sex without a condom and were therefore not supposed to bear children. This proscription of reproduction was based on fears of continued viral transmission and the potential spread of resistant virus as well as a concern for protecting the health of the seropositive woman and a fear that children born would either be HIV positive or orphaned. At that time, even patients on antiretroviral medication with suppressed viral loads were counseled to never have unprotected sex and to avoid pregnancy. This framing positioned people with AIDS and the associations as responsible for halting the transmission of the virus, again placing the burden of addressing the epidemic on its victims. Yet this notion of responsibility as voluntary infertility came into tension with a moral context in which individuals depended on social relationships for material survival. Living normal lives and fulfilling obligations to spouses and families meant successfully reproducing.[21]

In central Mozambique, bearing children is a sign of health, wealth, social status, and adult competence for both men and women, as reflected in the saying "he who has children needs nothing to be great."[22] One male association member explained to me: "You are not really a man without children. You can have a good job, lots of money, beautiful wife, but without kids, you are nothing." Though reproduction is socially important for both sexes, women disproportionately bear the burden and responsibility.[23] Infertility is frequently grounds for separation, but socially sanctioned polygamy protects men from this threat. In this context, voluntary infertility was tantamount to social suicide, particularly for women. The availability of ARVs complicated this issue further as healthy, HIV negative babies were being born to HIV positive mothers.

Associations in Chimoio were publicly criticized for preaching safe sex but tolerating pregnancies within the membership and even the leadership. These criticisms increased in response to the release of the most recent round of data that revealed an increase in national HIV prevalence. People living with HIV/AIDS were scapegoated for causing the increasing prevalence, and association members who were pregnant were singled out. There was also a grumbling, within and outside of the associations, that perhaps treatment was a mixed blessing in that it gave people the illusion of a cure and allowed them to deceive themselves and others about their serostatus. Debates about reproduction within the associations were divided along generational lines. Suraia, who had earlier shared with me how she first learned of AIDS, now indignantly told me:

> We are propagating the virus! If we would take this seriously, I think the prevalence would have already decreased. . . . We can't ourselves have life, rebirth, without this promise. I have another life. I've made that promise. I won't have sex without a condom. But I can see some people are destroying what we are trying to do in the associations. How can you come here and be pregnant? How? I feel bad for the youth, I do. At least, I have a child.

Embracing the spirit of individual responsibility, Suraia framed living positively as a tacit agreement to no longer reproduce, since that would spread the virus. Even while Suraia railed against association members spreading HIV, she acknowledged the predicament faced by those who were childless. Younger members, whose families often were not aware of their serostatus, asserted their right to have children and families of their own. Another association member, Clara, told me that she bore her HIV positive husband three children. She herself seroconverted during this process. When I asked why she consented to having sex without a condom if she knew he was positive and she was negative, she responded with exasperation:

> How would I get pregnant if we used a condom? I said to him, OK, you are like that, that's how it is. Aren't I a woman? Don't I want to give birth? We are married. Why would I use a condom if I wanted children?

She then shook her head and laughed at the implication that she should use a condom and not have children. In this case, Clara felt her social responsibility to bear children outweighed any individual responsibility to her health or to decrease transmission of the virus. Her narrative indicates she willingly accepted the risks of viral transmission, infection, and reinfection, though it begs the question of how much choice she really had to say no to the pressure to reproduce.

"IT IS BETTER TO BE WITH SOMEONE FROM THE ASSOCIATION. WHO ELSE CAN UNDERSTAND MY SITUATION?"

The stakes for condom use and disclosure were high. While many feared disclosure of HIV status could end a relationship with a seronegative partner, use of condoms could be interpreted as a lack of love and commitment.[24] Associations, therefore, offered members an important source of potential partners. Luiz first considered that he might have HIV in 1998, when a former lover approached him:

> I had a few lovers while in the military, and I knew three of them died, from this *doença prolongada*. One of my lovers came to me at the end, this was in 1998 or so, and she was really bad, very thin, and sores everywhere, hair falling out. She came to ask me for some money to help her get some clothes. I knew from then that I probably had it.

He was married and living with his family in a village on the Revue River when his wife gave birth but then fell ill. Luiz brought his wife to Chimoio, where the couple was diagnosed with HIV. Luiz's wife was told to stop breastfeeding in order to avoid infecting the infant. They returned to their families and informed her parents, who responded angrily, accusing him of infecting their daughter and publicly denouncing him. She left him, moving back in with her parents, and he left for Beira, where he found work selling *capulanas*, traveling the highway between Beira and Chimoio. He fell sick in 2003 as well, however, prompting him to seek care in the recently opened Day Hospital.

The next year, he began ARVs and his health improved. He began a relationship with a woman who lived near him.

> She wanted to stop using condoms. She saw that as an admirable thing. To speak of getting tested was an accusation. Why would I suggest such a thing? She said look, you can get a test and tell me the result. But I wanted us to be counseled together, so a third person could explain it all to her.

He never disclosed his status to her because he feared the angry response and public denouncement that he had suffered before:

> I couldn't tell her and she wouldn't go. I received food from the association, and she became suspicious. She said, "Don't people with AIDS receive food?" I began treatment and how could I hide it? Treatment my whole life and her not knowing?

He ended that relationship before he met Berta in the association:

> I began to think, this type of person, it's not worth it. She will harm me. It's better to find someone in my situation, whom I could tell everything to. If I told her, she might spread this news all around. It would ruin my life.

Similar to Luiz, Berta had had a previous marriage fall apart in the wake of HIV-related illness. She tested HIV positive and was advised to stop breastfeeding her six-month-old son. This caused considerable conflict in her husband's house:

> My father-in-law became suspicious. He said "why would you want to stop breastfeeding? Do you mean to kill our child?" Then my husband got sick too, and I was blamed for that.

Her son fell ill later that year and died, and Berta was thrown out of her husband's house. Luiz and Berta met in the association and had healthy twins. He explained:

> It was better to be with someone from the association. Who could better understand my situation? I get the medication for the two of us from the Day Hospital. There is nothing to hide with us. We really support each other. Being with a woman is a great help. If I am sick, who will take care of me? If she needs to take me to the hospital, she knows what to tell them.

While men such as Luiz tended to talk about the importance of being married in order to have a caregiving spouse, single women emphasized a desire to have children. Marta, a childless widow in her twenties, lamented:

> I am bitter because when I was told I had this problem [HIV], I was counseled that I could no longer have sexual relations without a condom. If I could have at least one child! But now, I am to suffer, childless. Who will care for me when my mother dies?

Many of the single women with children whom I spoke to said they had no plans to remarry, often reacting strongly, like Maria: "Marry again? *Chii*! Why would I go through that again? I have a son, I have my health, and I don't need to go looking for more trouble."

Those without children, however, often sought partners within associations. Hospital providers issued stern messages forbidding seropositive women to bear children. But in associations women found a middle ground between the rigid mandates of positive living, the realities of social norms, and the exigencies of survival that drove men and women to seek safe spaces for intimacy and support and to build families and future stability. Officially in the associations, members were discouraged from becoming pregnant, but as time went on, they were counseled to seek medical advice if they did decide to have children. Many spoke to me of their desire to find seropositive partners and have children when their CD4 count was high and their viral load suppressed.

A BREAK FROM THE PAST

The disparagement of African "backwardness" has a long history in Mozambique, from colonial times to socialist Frelimo, and continues in contemporary discourse and in the media, despite a current tendency of neoliberal reformers and government officials to idealize tradition.[25] This objectification of tradition is itself a product of Christianity's need for an antithesis in its struggle against sin. Tradition sets itself up against the Christian ways that have led to a neglect of customary practices.[26] The disparagement served as a rhetorical stance that positioned association members and those living positively as forward looking, educated, and worldly, aligned with the development and biomedical organizations who also blamed "African culture" for the high rates of HIV transmission and many of the complex, seemingly intractable problems of contemporary Africa, including the AIDS epidemic.[27] This culturalism diverts attention from the social, economic, and political origins of the HIV/AIDS epidemic and serves to blame the victims of the epidemic.[28]

While some, such as Elena, did manage to access robust forms of support through their biological status, thus illustrating the dynamics of what medical anthropologist Vinh-Kim Nguyen has characterized as therapeutic citizenship, hers was an exceptional case, particularly as the scale-up progressed and the numbers on treatment grew.[29] Other exceptions include the help Tomas received after breaking the silence and being thrown out of his mother's house;

in Tomas's case, a national AIDS organization helped him find a house and work, and he remained a committed activist. Elena also benefited from food supplementation and employment, and she managed to secure support for her siblings by registering them as "orphans and vulnerable children" (OVC) with a local NGO. Elena's success as an activist in Takashinga led to her recruitment to work in the Day Hospital as an adherence counselor during the expansion of treatment and eventually to full-time employment in the NHS. In the months following Florência's conversion, she was also hired to work as an adherence counselor in the local Day Hospital and thus earned access not only to life-saving antiretrovirals but also to the even scarcer but no less life-sustaining benefit of the AIDS economy, employment. The majority of people in treatment in central Mozambique, even those who sought membership in the associations, however, struggled to rebuild their lives while on ARVs, despite the *Vida Positiva* discourse that sought to normalize the disease. Many who converted to *Vida Positiva* were disappointed that, in the face of continued politico-economic marginalization, their observances and behavioral changes were not rewarded, and they experienced this as a violation of the moral economy. Associations themselves struggled with this dynamic. Association leaders, faced with the impossibility of providing benefits to all, deflected the notion that associations were places to seek material benefits. Gonçalo told members of his association:

> Yes, here sometimes opportunities appear, but that's not what the association is about. The purpose of the association is not to arrange employment! Others think the association is the place to be given food to eat! These are occasional and unexpected things!

His statement points to the tensions within the associations between the positive living orientation encouraging individual responsibility and self-care and the fact that most people came to associations seeking employment and material benefits. This tension led to frustration in both members and leaders and to an ever-greater emphasis on self-care. Yet calls for solidarity, friendship, and togetherness came into conflict with the inability of many associations to adequately address the material concerns of all their members.

THE ELUSIVENESS OF THERAPEUTIC CITIZENSHIP

During a conversation we had in 2004, when Elena was reflecting on her role in Takashinga and all that she had learned, she told me: "I thank the association and even HIV. I have travelled, to Dondo, Zimbabwe, to many places." She was referring to seminars and exchanges she had been a part of that took her around Mozambique and over the border to Zimbabwe. By expressing gratitude for this feared illness, she emphasized how far she had come and her embrace of *Vida Positiva*. She added: "When someone takes the test, they are left without doubts, happy, they could do something positive. People have fear, of what? It's for your health!" Elena had recovered her own health and had become a caregiver to countless others. She received food supplements from the association and also sent her young siblings through school, with NGO assistance for OVC. The greatest benefit seemed to be getting recruited to work in the Day Hospital, then as a regular employee of the NHS after the Day Hospital closed and HIV/AIDS care was integrated into the broader health system. Elena was able to build a house for her siblings and another one for herself thanks to her employment.

In many ways, Elena's case serves as an exemplar of what was possible in the AIDS economy. But her case is so exceptional that it also points to the elusiveness of those benefits, as well as to the inequality and exclusions of therapeutic citizenship. Associations of people living with HIV/AIDS were key nodes in the AIDS economy, where calls for solidarity were made amid fierce competition for resources. While associations were portrayed as spaces of dialogue and support, unauthorized testimonials about hunger, sex, and reproduction were marginalized, highlighting the rigid moralism of positive living. Performances of positive living obscured structural factors and resulted in blaming the victim when things did not go well. While these practices created a shared narrative, the focus on individual responsibility and morality served to silence many of those who struggled. Biomedical and public health education, oriented toward risk prevention, healthy choices, and individual behavioral change, joined development concepts of empowerment and participation in the discourse and practice of positive living. The individual focus of positive living and the Pentecostal notions of self-transformation reinforced a moralism that was just as often used to divide as it was to unite. Associations reinforced the atomizing tendencies of the AIDS treatment process, as the elusive rewards of the AIDS economy depended on the mercurial and scarce funding and support of development and global health organizations.

Antiretrovirals, associations, and *Vida Positiva* offered a way to commute the once certain social and biological death sentence of AIDS in Mozambique. The HIV diagnosis granted entry into a growing pool of fellow sufferers who could compete for the limited material benefits available to them. The one guarantee they had, if they were able to overcome the considerable obstacles to initiate treatment in the Day Hospital, was the promise of ARVs and the possibility of a few more years of life. The biosociality of the associations rested as much on the availability of food and material resources as on the disease diagnosis. The social networks emerging around HIV/AIDS depended on development institutions and biomedical technologies, leading to a kind of biomedicalized civil society, an economy of salvation that was often entwined with and at times in opposition to burgeoning Pentecostal religious movements. Those outside of the AIDS networks did not qualify for these benefits, while those within them faced the grim prospects of starving while on ARVs.

For some—Elena, Florência, Suraia, Luiz, Diogo, and others—associations were a space for learning, growth, opportunity, and solidarity. Yet for others, such as Rita and Joaquim, the competition and hierarchies within associations fostered jealousy, resentment, and distress, and many others were kept out altogether. When I asked Suzana, the activist discussed in the introduction who introduced me to a women's support group, to share her experiences with me, to tell me if she felt there was a sense of solidarity among those who were HIV positive, she explained that associations see other associations as rival political parties, competing for a limited amount of resources. HIV status was jealously guarded in the association. When three young women showed up interested in joining the association, which they had heard was distributing food and jobs, they were asked to produce their papers from the hospital. When they could not, they were literally chased out by the jeering crowd. This may be indicative of HIV interventions that separated people into categories, and in this atmosphere of scarcity and competition, turned on each other. Scarcity can transform the associations, potential spaces for solidarity, into venues for competition, examples of Primo Levi's "Grey Zones": "morally ambiguous spaces . . . where survival imperatives overcome human solidarity as individuals jockey desperately for a shred of advantage."[30] This scarcity is a result of thirty years of austerity measures imposed by the IMF, which have restricted the funding available for health, education, and poverty reduction and have not led to improved livelihoods for the majority. Instead, Mozambique continues to favor natural resource extraction "mega-projects," including aluminum, minerals, coal, natural gas, and oil, largely run by transnational corporations, as well as export-oriented agriculture such as tobacco and cashew nuts.[31] These policies have resulted in an increase in GDP but few jobs. Growth has been concentrated among the top 10 percent of wage earners and beyond this has generated wealth for a very small, elite group. Over the 2000s, the incomes of the wealthiest households in Mozambique increased while the incomes of the poorest households decreased.[32] Viewed from this structural perspective, the scarcity and competition within associations has resulted not from a lack of resources but from a lack of distribution of existing resources and a systematic disinvestment in poor communities mandated by structural adjustment policies. In such a context, AIDS treatment interventions that narrowly focused on individual biology and behavior and ignored the broader, collective conditions of survival fostered competition and resentment.

4 "We Can't Find This Spirit of Help"

THE USES OF COMMUNITY LABOR

The early grassroots responses to AIDS in southeastern Africa drew heavily on voluntary labor, "a force of largely female religious charity and community spirit."[1] These efforts would come to be called community home-based care (CHBC). UNAIDS recognized these volunteers as "key pillars" of AIDS treatment programs.[2] Arminda, like other CHBC volunteers, visited chronically ill individuals in Chimoio's *bairros* to educate them and their families about HIV, offering comfort-oriented basic care as well as emotional and spiritual support and referral to appropriate health and social services. Arminda worked with Mufudzi, a Christian organization that would become the exemplar for Mozambique's CBHC scale-up.

Arminda described her work to me during the early period of the AIDS treatment scale-up:

> I began visiting Beatriz five months ago. When I first arrived, Beatriz would go to the clinic one day, make an appointment, then follow other programs [i.e., go to *n'angas*], but she remained sick.

During these visits, Arminda assisted with daily activities and provided spiritual and emotional support. When Beatriz's daughter also became sick, Arminda asked Beatriz's husband: "Will you accept, starting today, your wife accompanies us, begins new consultations?" Arminda was asking permission to take Beatriz to get tested for HIV. Arminda also spoke about this with Beatriz's father, who then spoke with his son-in-law. As a CHBC volunteer, Arminda navigated complex family dynamics in counseling ill individuals and their families, recruiting them for HIV testing, and accompanying them through treatment. The family agreed to let Arminda take Beatriz to the testing center. Arminda took Beatriz, along with another young woman, Lídia, and Lídia's husband. "They were all positive, and he also had tuberculosis" Arminda explained and added, "Now they are all following their treatment. I keep visiting them, checking on them, but they are fine. Just Beatriz's husband, he doesn't want to test, but his wife, she is free to pursue her treatment and he has no problem with us."

This chapter tracks the intertwined biographies of CHBC, Arminda, and the organization she worked for, Mufudzi. My focus is on Arminda and the experiences, aspirations, skills, and values she brought to her work as a volunteer, as well as the ways her own life converged with the rise and fall of the organization that pioneered CHBC in this region and with the scale-up. The initial model of CHBC, begun in the mid-1990s, had a pragmatic, palliative, and spiritual orientation toward relieving suffering and addressing material deprivation. Mufudzi recruited "motherly" women, who were considered wise, capable of maintaining confidentiality, and gifted at confronting suffering and death gracefully and compassionately. Volunteers—nonprofessionals grounded in the local logics of care—were oriented toward the material and spiritual needs of their patients. They drew on Pentecostal and biomedical practices that emphasized individual and collective well-being and explicitly pointed to civilization and self-improvement to distinguish themselves and their worldview from the *n'angas*. Following the arrival of rapid HIV testing and anti-retroviral treatment in the early 2000s, CHBC was scaled up when a MISAU working group incorporated Mufudzi's approach into what became the national CHBC model. As the only CHBC organization operated and run by non-health-care professionals in Mozambique, Mufudzi was the exemplar for the scale-up. At the same time, a concern that volunteers were "just praying" led the working group to focus on establishing "minimum quality standards" for technically oriented care, such as adherence to medications, tuberculosis screening, and management of opportunistic infection prophylaxis. As a consequence of the scale-up, CHBC returned to Mufudzi through standardized protocols and increased donor funding that catalyzed changes. The rapid pace and the technical orientation of the scale-up altered the practice of CHBC by de-emphasizing attention to basic needs such as food and more narrowly defining "care" as technically oriented work.

This chapter emphasizes Arminda's singular experience to highlight the aspirations and frustrations of the CHBC volunteers who made up the social infrastructure of the AIDS treatment interventions.[3] Caught between professionalization and preservation of the "volunteer spirit," the volunteers were trapped in a marginal position and were ultimately excluded from the intervention despite the key role they played in initiating the program.[4] A gendered division of labor anchored the volunteers' marginal position. The volunteers were locally referred to as *mães*, Portuguese for "mothers." Care, particularly the nontechnical aspects conducted within households, is marked as a woman's activity and marginalized within a global political economy organized around technology as a driver of improved health.[5] While the community embeddedness and dedication of the volunteers was seen as a strength by MISAU, the desire to monitor and regulate the care via standardized clinical protocols rendered the untrained and semiliterate volunteers as suspect, potentially harmful, and in need of supervision. Locally marked in this way, the volunteers had a tenuous connection to the global space of the scale-up, demarcated by biomedical expertise and the discourse of transnational biomedical technology.[6]

Arminda and many of her CHBC colleagues felt abandoned, despite their work having served as the vanguard and national model for CHBC. The labor of the volunteers was exploited as a resource, made freely available by widespread underemployment, to be extracted in the name of cost-effectiveness. This chapter considers how this happened and in doing so raises questions about the underlying values of global health interventions and the communities they constitute through interventions such as the AIDS treatment scale-up.

MUFUDZI AND THE EMERGENCE OF COMMUNITY HOME-BASED CARE

Mufudzi (Shepherd) was founded in 1995 through a partnership between the faith-based Zimbabwean Muchengeti (Care Giver) and a faith-based European NGO working in Zimbabwe. These organizations were working to support repatriation of Mozambican refugees who had fled to Zimbabwe during the war but now could return home. With HIV/AIDS already a major issue in Zimbabwe, they wanted to mobilize Mozambican churches with ties to congregations across the border around HIV/AIDS. These partners found eight Mozambican churches (four Pentecostal, three mainstream Protestant, and one Catholic) willing to work with them. They formed Mufudzi, which would become one of the principal NGOs active in central Mozambique in community-based HIV/AIDS interventions. Mufudzi was an independent organization that operated through its member churches and individual volunteers who did not have to belong to member churches or be Christian.

One of Mufudzi's founding members recalled the challenges of organizing around HIV in the mid-1990s:

> The initial reception [in the churches] was difficult because the pastors didn't accept this word, HIV/AIDS. They thought those with AIDS were people with immoral lives and not people in the church. It wasn't relevant to them. We kept working on educating them, until we encountered the story of a pastor who got sick and died of HIV/AIDS. That alerted the pastors that HIV/AIDS doesn't distinguish amongst churches or morality.

In this recollection, HIV/AIDS was not understood as a relevant priority to some of these churches until it could be made visible in a more immediate way. One way it could be made visible was by "giving AIDS a face" and showing that the disease could affect the members of one's own church community and was not restricted to the immoral "other."

Another way HIV was made visible and relevant was by creating opportunities linked to education about HIV or care for people with AIDS, such as a meal; remunerative labor; or opportunities for training, education, service, and recognition: "People were just coming out of the war and were eager to learn anything. They came to the trainings partly to get a meal, but as they learned about HIV, people became really interested. They said: 'We have these problems here.'" As with "therapeutic congregations" (i.e., the associations discussed in chapter 3 that were formed to support HIV positive members), interventions often represented opportunities for material support, and this was central to the AIDS economy in the treatment scale-up.

CHBC was one of Mufudzi's first initiatives.[7] Muchengeti ran a CHBC program in Mutare, located near the Mozambican border in Zimbabwe, and Mufudzi adapted that program's Shona-language materials for its own use. Mufudzi's CHBC program was explicitly based on the model of pastoral visits that many local churches already engaged in: visiting ailing parishioners and offering support, including help with household work, material assistance, and prayer. The difference was that Mufudzi visited people irrespective of church affiliation and was oriented toward caring for people with AIDS and other chronic diseases.[8]

Arminda was part of Mufudzi's first volunteer cohort and remained a volunteer throughout my research. She grew up in a village liberated by Frelimo during the war of independence against Portugal in the 1960s. Her village was targeted in Renamo's initial insurgency in the late 1970s:

> We suffered the war out there in the bush, the war of our neighbor Ian Smith [Rhodesian prime minister]. He came with airplanes, dropping bombs. We ran carrying bundles in our hands, whatever we could fit on our heads. I was a girl at the time but my mother was pregnant, so I had to carry my baby brother.

Arminda's family fled to neighboring Zimbabwe as the conflict escalated. She settled in Chimoio after the cease-fire and lived with her daughters behind the market stall she operated. Arminda became an active member of the Universal Church of the Kingdom of God, an international Pentecostal church, soon after she moved to Chimoio in the mid-1990s, when she saw her daughter's persistent illness successfully healed by prayer in this church. She recalled first hearing about Mufudzi as "this organization where many people come together from different countries. They get together and exchange opinions . . . about civilization, how to live with others religiously. I said, I think I could benefit from that." It reminded her of an association she had been part of as a refugee in Zimbabwe:

> We had a partnership there, we contributed and then there was help for all in times of illness or death. We also studied ideas together. . . . [Mufudzi] could help me like that association from Zimbabwe did. So I liked it and entered that first training. It was about how to do business, to help orphans, the sick, how to help people . . . that was my motivation, religious union, about life, studying about these positive diseases.

As this passage indicates, Arminda had multiple motivations to become a volunteer, including opportunities to enact pro-social, altruistic, civic, and spiritual service. These motivations existed alongside her desire for education and self-improvement. The Mufudzi organization, supported by Zimbabwean and European colleagues, was part of the emerging global fight against AIDS and based on regionally circulating CHBC models. Volunteering with Mufudzi promised Arminda proximity to a cosmopolitanism that the Zimbabwean association and her own church represented. By joining Mufudzi, Arminda was placing herself on a "forward moving trajectory."[9] Arminda proudly displayed the certificates she had earned in her training as tangible evidence of this progress of her own "civilization." These represented her ambivalence toward "tradition," as the high prevalence of HIV has been attributed to ignorance as well as various "traditional" practices and beliefs.[10] Indeed, CHBC leadership tended to have formal theological training and frowned on AICs and *profetes* as pagan. They blamed *n'angas* and *profetes* for making the epidemic worse by spreading falsehoods about HIV; preventing people from seeking biomedical care; tolerating polygamy, which for the CHBC leadership amounted to adultery; and generally promoting ignorant practices. Some pastors who served as leaders in Mufudzi saw the education and conversion of members of AICs as a part of their mission to fight HIV/AIDS so that they might leave their so-called backward and ignorant ways behind. Several pastors and *profetes* of AICs with whom I spoke understood this as Mufudzi's mission, viewed Mufudzi's work with suspicion, and refused to engage with their HIV/AIDS outreach efforts.

ARMINDA, MUFUDZI, AND CHBC:
"PRAYER IS MEDICINE"

The first Mufudzi group of twenty-eight volunteers consisted of women in their forties or fifties deemed to be "good in caring, not afraid of cleaning or of intimacy with those who were sick and dying, who really were motherly," according to one of the founders. Half were literate. They had been identified by their churches as "wise, able to maintain confidentiality, strong in faith, and wanting to do the work without pay. It was more of a calling, a biblical mandate." This was a defining aspect of CHBC that Mufudzi leadership maintained throughout the intervention: volunteers needed to be motivated by altruism rather than personal gain, and therefore the work needed to be freely given rather than remunerated.[11] This stance would become a source of tension between Mufudzi funders, MISAU, and volunteers as the landscape of HIV care was transformed by the scale-up, but it was not an issue at this early stage when there was little money available. When the project began in the mid-1990s, the task of the volunteers was to provide palliative care and support to people who were facing imminent death, if not actively dying. Volunteers and health-care providers recalled overwhelmed hospital staff sending people home to die, telling their family members there was nothing more to be done. Volunteers spoke of the need to bring compassion and dignity to people who felt abandoned.

Volunteers attended a two-week workshop on CHBC focused on HIV transmission, the signs of AIDS, and how to care for an HIV-positive, often bedbound person at home. This included assessing for dehydration, malnutrition, fever, and open wounds and bedsores; bathing the person and washing bedclothes; and basic physical therapy. Alongside this bodily care were techniques for counseling and educating about HIV, as well as spiritual support. The CHBC volunteers worked in the neighborhoods in which they lived. They visited all chronically ill individuals in a neighborhood to educate them and their families about HIV, offering comfort-oriented basic care as well as emotional and spiritual support and referral to appropriate health and social services. The neighborhood political leaders, the *secretários dos bairros*, informed volunteers of new cases of illness, and volunteers also identified cases on their own. If ill individuals and their families accepted their care and invited them back, volunteers would work with them over time. Volunteers were officially assigned up to five or six patients to attend to, but in practice they might accompany many more than that.

I met many of Arminda's patients. One of them, Severino, recounted his history with Arminda. He recalled, "When I first got sick, I was in a lot of pain whenever I awoke, difficulty breathing, diarrhea, headache, no strength." He went to a clinic, but this was prior to the treatment scale-up. They did not resolve the problem. He recounted trips to *n'angas*, "one near the Pungwe River, several hours away, a good healer, not like these in the city. He gave me something that helped, but after a while it stopped working, so I went to another one, near Vanduzi, who explained my ancestors were attacking me because I had not shown them proper respect. I followed his instructions, and again, I got better, but again, I had a relapse. I saw another *n'anga* in Tete, another in Zobue at the border with Malawi." He also saw a private biomedical practitioner, a nurse in his neighborhood who gave him injections. Then he bought medicines in the market, but "always the same, I'd be better for a short while but then relapse."

Severino described how Arminda began to visit, after all these attempts at recovery had failed: "I was living alone. I was at zero. I was sick and had nothing and felt I'd tried everything. She'd come by, and when I was well, I'd visit her as well." It was only after they had developed a relationship that Arminda asked, "Have you gone to the Day Hospital?" Severino told her, "I tried to get there the year before last. But they said no, you have to get tested first, for HIV." He went on to explain, "So I went to get tested, but they said I had to go to the hospital first. Now I was getting confused. I speak Portuguese well, but reading, I'm not so good. All these doors, papers, places to go. I just went home. And that was it." Arminda picked him up the next day, and they went together. Severino describes Arminda as his "guide" and "savior": "I think she saved me. When I had nowhere to turn and nothing to eat, she took me to the proper place, and I received food and the treatment I needed. I am much better now, working more, eating more." In this way CHBC volunteers entered into the kinship networks that guide a sick person from one source of treatment to another in the "quest for therapy" in much of Africa.[12]

Arminda helped her patients navigate the confusing health-care system and the many steps required to access life-saving ARVs. Another of Arminda's patients had similarly received visits from Arminda over a long period of time. This woman only went to get tested after her husband died. She told me of Arminda, "This woman saved me, because of this woman, I'm fine." She encouraged others to go to Arminda as well: "I tell them, go to her, she that accompanied me. Arminda cures!" Anthropologist John Janzen, working in what was then Zaire, termed such networks "therapy management groups." He noted they emerged in a colonial context where indigenous healers were outlawed and driven underground and there was little public health infrastructure available for colonial subjects.[13]

Entering into these networks was a form of labor, uncompensated and unprotected. Arminda described the risks she took in one situation in which her involvement with a family resulted in threats on her life:

> One girl who lives nearby, she lost her first child. She became pregnant again, lost this child as well. She was sick, and she thought maybe the problem was with her husband. So she came and spoke to me, I spoke with her and her husband, and encouraged them to go to the hospital, to take that test.

Only the woman got tested. The result was positive, and she was told to bring her husband to get tested as well. But her husband wanted nothing to do with it. Arminda explained to me how precarious the pregnant woman's situation was now. The husband stopped visiting Arminda and blamed the wife for all their troubles. "He hit her and she came running to me for help. She came here, bleeding. I asked her what happened, and she told me her husband threw her out, saying 'go to the house of that lady. Go to the house of she who accompanied you and stay there.'" They went to the police, who asked for the husband to come see them. That husband said that if he were to be detained by the police, he would "burn her parent's house as well as the house of the activist, me!" So Arminda told me the woman stopped everything. "It ended there." The woman and her husband separated. By entering into the highly charged terrain of illness, diagnosis, and treatment, where a diagnosis might be understood as an accusation of impropriety and sickness was often seen to be sent by angry ancestors or jealous rivals, volunteers like Arminda ran the risk of offending the very people they were trying to help.

In Arminda's telling, her own biography led her into the work. She had experience caring for a daughter and a brother with AIDS. She recalled what she had inherited and learned from her father, who was a healer: "I have a personal spirit for this. My father was a *n'anga*. He had a lot of patience. I remember a boy who came with a problem in his spinal column and we massaged him every morning. . . . Sick people always came." Arminda noted that their house was always full of people. She told me that doing this work was not difficult for her because of this:

> It's not difficult for me, because in my father's house, we always ate together [patients and family]. We were all one family. Now, I don't know if this is the spirit I have, but I think for me, this is normal. I once asked "*Papá*, why is our family always so full? My uncle's house is not like this. Why is ours?" He answered, "when you are accustomed to hosting guests in your home, at another moment, you will find yourself in another country, another place, and those you helped will recognize you and open their homes."

Arminda took pride in the trust that her neighbors granted her by opening up to her about their HIV status and their personal challenges. The ill and their family members sought her out: "They say, '*Mamá*, I can tell you my secret'" (see figure 14). In other cases, Arminda would gradually approach families, taking her time to familiarize herself with the situation and to gain their trust. Arminda gained status in her community and was pleased she could carry on the spirit of her father's work, interpreting her father's guidance to mean her own generosity would be repaid in a moral economy where, in the words of anthropologist Sasha Newell, "social relationships take priority. . . . [T]he maintenance and accumulation of

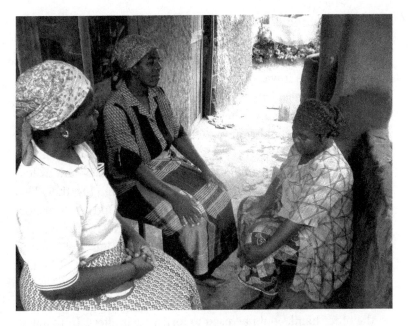

Figure 14. Arminda (left) consulting with fellow CHBC volunteers who live nearby.

these relationships is its own kind of profit."[14] Volunteers saw their work as being therapeutic not only on an individual but also on a communal level.

One common saying among both volunteers and patients was "prayer is medicine." In keeping with local Pentecostal church practices, volunteers prayed for God or the Holy Spirit to directly intercede and heal. Arminda liked to begin visits with a prayer, but she took care to ask permission before initiating one. The patient and all family members present were invited to join hands and participate. She noted, "There could be a demon in that house that wants to kill." In such cases, Arminda explained, "First I get the Lord's blessing that he may help me, bring me strength, intelligence. It's not luck; it's not knowledge: without the Lord in my heart, I would get upset, leave, but with the power of the Lord, I win those people over and take them to the hospital." These notions of spirits acting in the world are characteristic of contemporary African Pentecostal churches and are widely shared in Chimoio, and this was just as much a statement of world views as it was of therapeutics.[15] Though divination in the realm of ancestral spirits and sorcery (*uroi*) was perceived as backward and pagan, Arminda herself never disputed the power of the *n'anga*. Arminda would contrast Christian prayer with the *n'anga's* divination: "The *n'anga* will say that person did this, that person will be accused." Church members frequently felt these accusations fostered conflict, while they felt prayer brought people together. This was reflected in another phrase volunteers used: "God sends misfortune so that people may be united." Christian notions of forgiveness, charity, and attention to the less fortunate were thus mobilized to address guilt and blame within individuals and families. Arminda also repeated clinicians' warnings that the *n'anga's* herbal treatments should not be taken with medication, and noted that prayer, on the other hand, could be used to fortify their effect. In this way, Arminda and many in Mufudzi and in the AIDS economy aligned Christian approaches with biomedicine and against *n'angas*.

Though volunteers had faith in the power of prayer, this faith was accompanied by a concern for basic needs. Volunteers consistently pointed to poverty and hunger as the principal challenges their patients faced as they shared their stories with each other. While recounting the history of the CHBC program, volunteers recalled that they were ashamed of visiting sick people empty-handed. They began bringing their patients small amounts of food from their own homes, until Mufudzi obtained a contract with the WFP to provide food (discussed later in this chapter). This notably improved the success volunteers had in recruiting patients. As one of the early coordinators recalled: "Families hid their sick at first . . . but they opened their doors for food." Food was conceived as a family and communal intervention as much as for an individual's health. One volunteer explained that if a sick person can "bring benefits" to the entire family, they would be more likely to unite the family around them.

In the early years of CHBC, volunteers focused on palliative and comfort-oriented care, education, and improving basic health and relationships through a diverse set of techniques and approaches, including bodily care, prayer, food, help with domestic chores, compassion, and counseling. While spiritual motivations were part of the community labor of volunteers, they cited opportunities for service, education, and self-improvement as additional motivating factors.[16] They also hoped that their efforts would bring them stable employment, recognition and appreciation, and compensation, particularly as the treatment scale-up brought unprecedented resources to Mufudzi and other NGOs working on HIV/AIDS issues.

MUFUDZI'S SCALE-UP

Mufudzi was well-positioned to benefit from the treatment scale-up. In the early 2000s, CHBC was a UNAIDS Best Practice already implemented in much of southern and eastern Africa. MISAU convened a working group on CHBC to develop a national plan that included members of government and national and international NGOs. Mufudzi was officially a part of the working group, but its participation was limited to email contact, as there was no funding to transport anyone from Chimoio, a flight or full day's drive from the location of the working group meetings in Maputo, the country's capital, located in southeastern Mozambique. The best-known CHBC programs operating in the country were Mufudzi in Chimoio and a nurse-run intervention based in Maputo. Mufudzi became the model for the national program because it was community based and designed for lay volunteers. At the same time, however, there were concerns that, in the words of one working group member, volunteers "were just praying, and a lot more could be done, even without ARVs, to prolong life and make people more comfortable and less stigmatized." A national CHBC manual was created that was based on Mufudzi's, but Mufudzi members were upset that spiritual components of care, prominent in their version, were nearly absent in the national manual. Nonetheless, MISAU encouraged organizations interested in starting CHBC programs to visit Mufudzi and learn from their approach. Volunteers became accustomed to frequent visits from MISAU officials and AIDS organizations from around the country.

CHBC was given a central role in the initial model for HIV/AIDS treatment services scale-up in Mozambique, termed the Integrated Health Network. According to MISAU's national HIV/AIDS strategy manual, "the link between the HIV/AIDS clinic and home-based care is the cornerstone for the monitoring and treatment of PLWHA [People Living with HIV/AIDS]."[17] As medications became available, CHBC shifted from palliative care to recruiting individuals for testing and supporting ARV initiation and maintenance. The focus on treatment also shifted the framing of care in an increasingly technical direction. In its definition of CHBC, the MISAU distinguished between "home-based care" and "home visits":

> "Care" is defined as the attention provided at home to PLWHA and their families, which includes . . . adherence to drugs and a referral system between the National Health Services and the community . . . while home "visits" generally have social, emotional and spiritual support as their objective.[18]

Care was defined as an activity with a technical orientation relating to a biomedical conception of health and disease and that involved referral and connection to biomedical services.[19] Visits that were not technically oriented were simply home visits and did not qualify as home-based care. The working group concern that volunteers were "just praying" can be read into these definitions, as social, emotional, and spiritual support did not constitute care. Though Mufudzi's community orientation made it the favored initial model, national certification courses were taught by nurses, and the official CHBC training manual doubled in size between 2002 and 2006, from 83 to 160 pages, to accommodate increasing amounts of technical information.

Volunteers had always collected data for Mufudzi and funders. The national data collection form, which had both words and pictures for the many illiterate volunteers, required a new level of detail.[20] The data were pooled at the organization level and "uploaded" to the MISAU and donors. The 2006 version included number of visits, death, loss to follow-up, enrollment in antiretroviral or tuberculosis treatment, and designation of a range of issues that required various referrals: to the Day Hospital, to supplemental food support, to education for children, legal issues, the presence of orphans in the household, and inadequate income. By 2010, the data collection form was more clinical, abandoning the original sense of "care" in favor of a biomedical definition.[21] Care categories focused on enrollment in antiretroviral and tuberculosis treatment, use of antibiotic prophylaxis, pregnancy, enrollment in the Day Hospital, loss to follow-up, and death. Dropped from the earlier version were the majority of "social" categories, including supplemental food support and income.

As the treatment scale-up proceeded, there was more emphasis on monitoring, evaluation, and accountability, which created increasing amounts of required documentation. Volunteers were asked to master complex domains of knowledge that the expanding training module encompassed and to perform more formal documentation procedures.[22] These changes led to the establishment of minimum qualifications for volunteers: six years of schooling and the ability to read and write. In effect, this shifted the profile from the older, "motherly" individual Mufudzi sought to a more educated, younger profile that MISAU preferred.[23] Not only was the work of the CHBC uncompensated, the lack of compensation was now justified by sidelining the kind of holistic care the CHBC volunteers provided.

Scale-up incorporated CHBC into the Integrated Health Network and made more resources available for the intervention. Though the national program was modeled on Mufudzi's, changes introduced at a national level pushed CHBC in a more technical direction, which would have mixed impacts on Mufudzi's volunteers, as they were increasingly told their skill set was obsolete by officials from MISAU and partner organizations. In tandem with this technicization, the massive infusion of resources would also have an impact on Mufudzi and CHBC volunteers.

SHIFTING LANDSCAPES OF CARE AND THE PROFESSIONALIZATION OF MUFUDZI

Mufudzi increased and expanded in step with the scale-up. A formal organization structure with a constitution and a governing assembly were established. The first salaried positions were created in 1999, for the director; chief administrator; and heads of the CHBC, pastor education, and youth programs. The professional staff grew to as many as fifty-six, only four of whom had been founding members. An initial budget of just over US$600, spent on training and renting a shared office space, mushroomed in the 2000s to US$10,000 and then US$700,000. The larger quantities of funding came from PEPFAR, through a partnership with a locally operating American NGO. More than eighty churches became members, and the scale of activities similarly expanded. There were as many as 130 CHBC volunteers in Chimoio, and 240 for the five districts of the province, as programs were initiated throughout the region. Mufudzi moved from a borrowed back room to rented office space in the early 2000s. Mufudzi built its own office in 2008. Mufudzi expanded its activities to include the association of people living with HIV/AIDS with over seven hundred registered members, Takashinga, and programs for OVC.[24] This increased funding stoked discontent over who received payment and who did not, which ultimately led to the marginalization of a significant number of volunteers.

With the rapid treatment scale-up leading to a growing number of CHBC organizations, MISAU recommended an incentive rate of 60 percent of the minimum wage (amounting to about US$24/month) for volunteers, with maximum allowable payment not to exceed the minimum wage.[25] According to a working group participant, the consensus within the group was that poor women caring for others deserved to be paid something. The recommendation was also meant to prevent one particularly well-resourced NGO from paying volunteers higher salaries than nurses and then triggering a "brain drain" from the public sector to NGOs.[26]

Payment was a controversial issue within Mufudzi. In the mid-1990s, nobody was paid for working with people with HIV, and most Mufudzi members indeed said they started the work without the expectation of payment. They did, however, hope their training, certifications, and connection to the NGO networks might lead to employment opportunities. As the scale-up progressed and the amount of money available nationally for HIV/AIDS exponentially increased and was channeled into Mufudzi, the assumption the volunteers would not be paid remained, even as the organization professionalized. Volunteers, however, began requesting their share of the funding, particularly when a second NGO in Chimoio began providing CHBC modeled on Mufudzi's practice and provided its volunteers the incentive. At one meeting, a salaried program coordinator scolded the volunteers who raised this issue:

> This work should come from the heart. It should not be done for payment, but to help our neighbors, our brothers and sisters. It is our work that we do. If we get paid, it is not a bad thing, but we do not do this work in order to be paid, and we do the work even when we are not being paid.

Mufudzi's administrators feared that payments would distort the work and attract opportunists who would be less effective than those motivated by altruism and a religious calling. Most of those who objected to paying CHBC volunteers had salaried positions themselves, however. The emphasis on a moral and spiritual calling distracted from the fact that there was now money being made in the AIDS economy, but little of it was reaching the volunteers.

Not only were CHBC workers not paid for their work, they needed continued material support in order to be able to successfully perform that work. Volunteers also felt they were not well supported with the necessary resources to carry out their duties. A patient "might not have food," Arminda explained, so "you have to bring him food. But that is more than Mufudzi even provides us for ourselves." Arminda emphasized that CHBC volunteers did not feel they were given adequate supplies to perform their work:

> What if the patient cannot walk? I have to get in that *chapa* with him and pay for it. With what money do I do that? I had a patient whose family would not touch his soiled clothing. I showed them how to wash it without fear of contamination. I have to help clean him, with what soap? I can't wash the entire neighborhood with my own soap. This work takes patience, feeling, and courage.

Still, volunteers strove to provide appropriate and quality care through the changes. As the scale-up proceeded, however, the assessments of those around them changed. In 2003, an expatriate administrator of an NGO that worked with Mufudzi told me: "I think it's horrible to pay church women to visit their neighbors when they are sick. Shouldn't they just do so because it's the right thing to do?" Her comment seemed to conflate the form of humanitarian volunteering engaged in by relatively affluent expatriates who chose to do so for limited periods of time with the labor that poor, local women engaged in for many years in Chimoio.

When MISAU changed the guidelines and began recommending a monetary incentive of 60 percent of the minimum wage, Mufudzi attempted to meet that through group rather than individual incentives and experimented with a microcredit project and a community garden for volunteers, but the benefits were not well distributed among the volunteers, and nothing was sustained. Arminda recounted how when she first began, there was no payment, but as they expanded, they began to receive nonmonetary incentives. WHO and MISAU guidelines encouraged these incentives: refresher training and exchanges with other groups, during which volunteers were provided with snacks and lunches; certificates;

organization T-shirts; *capulanas*; and annual bonuses of rice, corn, oil, or soap.

Finally, in 2008, under pressure from Mufudzi's CHBC funder to provide volunteers their incentives and in response to increasing frustration from the volunteers, it was agreed that volunteers would be paid the recommended amount, but the number of CHBC volunteers was cut by 40 percent, as the available funding would only cover a limited number. According to a Mufudzi administrator, the funder would or could not support group payment schemes, such as funding a group microcredit project, and insisted on incentives for individual volunteers. When Arminda and a few other volunteers were finally awarded monetary incentives after several years of acrimony, the fact that nearly half of the volunteers were cut felt demoralizing. Those cut—older and less-educated volunteers—were invited to work with OVC, which did not provide monetary incentives. Most of these volunteers held out hope they might be reinstated to CHBC.

Still, the volunteers welcomed the changes that they could see resulted in improvements for their patients, even if these increased their workload. They desired training and education so did not protest the technical shift. They continued with the same approach, but worked to incorporate the increased clinical aspects and demands for referral and documentation. Those who could not read and write struggled with documentation but worked around it by recruiting literate colleagues and family members to help them. Neighborhood CHBC teams tried to have at least one literate member who organized documentation. Volunteers appreciated the closer connection with the health services and the increase in treatments their patients accessed. They did complain, however, about not being respected or treated well by clinical staff when they accompanied patients to the clinic. Another welcome change that the scale-up brought was a WFP contract, which provided monthly food baskets to patients, but this unfortunately became divisive when volunteers were told not to share the available food among all their patients, as had been their practice, but rather to target those receiving treatment. This produced resentment and jealousy among their patients. Many patients and their families accused volunteers of eating the food that was meant for them and of benefiting from their suffering.

Volunteers felt the shifting attitude and did complain about not being respected or treated well by clinical staff when they accompanied patients to the clinic. The comment "all they do is pray" was a frequent characterization of Mufudzi's CHBC program in the mid- to late 2000s by NGO and MISAU administrators and indicated that Mufudzi's CHBC no longer resembled "care" despite the fact that its practices were embedded in the national manual. A young official in the provincial health department with whom I discussed CHBC in 2010 even denied that Mufudzi had ever served as the model for CHBC, asking how illiterate and uneducated women could be expected to provide effective home-based care. These comments point not only to an overwhelmingly technical and clinical conception of care, but also to the ways community labor was gendered and naturalized, seen as something women should somehow "just do." While Mozambican CHBC began in Chimoio as a holistic intervention run by female church-based volunteers, it became technicized through the scale-up to the extent that the practices of the vanguard of CHBC were no longer recognizable to those implementing the scale-up. While the volunteers continued to be dedicated to their work, the landscape around them shifted considerably.

CHICA: "YES, I AM BETTER. BUT MY STOMACH HURTS!"

By 2010, Mufudzi was facing multiple organizational challenges. CHBC was no longer a top priority of the funding partner, which had changed to another international organization, and the emphasis in MISAU was now on providing treatment in the broader primary care system rather than through the integrated health network.

Community outreach and support, already marginal once treatment had arrived, was even less of a priority. Mufudzi would lose the majority of its CHBC funding that year, and its CHBC program would come to an end by 2012. I was in Chimoio in 2010 and accompanied Arminda on her visit to Chica, a woman whom she had recruited for testing and treatment. Arminda was concerned about Chica's difficulties adhering to her medications. We arrived at Chica's house around lunchtime. A young woman was cooking peas in front of the family hut as an elderly woman and two children ate *sadza* that was the characteristic beige color of USAID corn-soy blend. On the far side of the yard, another young woman and man sat selling a fermented sugarcane brew (*nipa*). We entered the hut. Arminda initiated the visit with a prayer and proudly introduced Chica, saying: "Here is my patient. I can tell you she is much better!" Chica added: "Yes, I am better. But my stomach hurts!"

In the months since Arminda had first seen her, Chica's health and appearance had improved significantly, despite spotty adherence and clinic attendance. Chica endorsed the characteristic hunger of ARVs: "If I take my pills at night, my stomach wakes me up, and I have to eat. In the morning when I awake, I have to eat again." She had been awarded a WFP ration card, entitling her to receive 10 kilograms of corn-soy blend and 1 kilogram of legumes per month, an amount that, when shared among her three children, two grandchildren, and elderly mother, lasted four days.[27] She also sold *nipa* and sought odd jobs. When she did not have food to eat, Chica skipped her ARVs. Arminda listened and discussed possible avenues of support. Chica disclosed that she engaged in serial short-lived sexual relationships with men who could provide her with material support and did not always use condoms. Her current stomach pain was accompanied by a foul-smelling vaginal discharge that she was ashamed to reveal to a clinician lest she be rebuked for having unprotected sex. She occasionally treated it with antibiotics, when she could afford to seek treatment. Arminda arranged to accompany Chica to the clinic later that week so she could be assessed and also encouraged her to stay adherent to her antiretro-virals. Arminda would visit daily for the rest of the week, bringing food from her own home for Chica to take with her ARVs. Many taking treatment pointed to this contradiction: that they struggled to feed themselves and their families even while they managed to obtain lifesaving pharmaceutical treatment. This persisted despite the dynamics illustrated by this case: that food insecurity may drive the spread of the HIV epidemic.

With a wrinkled brow, Arminda expressed mixed feelings follow-ing the visit:

> That's the difficulty of this work. When a patient doesn't have food, doesn't have soap to wash their clothes, no way of getting to the hos-pital when they are ill, with children who depend on her. . . . I bring them things from my own home, because I can't let a patient die of hunger. You have to take a bit of whatever you have. Sometimes she'll come herself to my house, "*Mamá*, I'm hungry!" But what can I do? I'm a person too.

Arminda felt obligated to offer whatever food she could as a gesture of solidarity and recognition of Chica's suffering and her need. She and her fellow volunteers were acutely aware of their limitations, and they were often overwhelmed by the needs of their patients. While they experienced considerable satisfaction when their patients recovered, they were distressed by their inability to address their patients' basic needs, especially food. They also endured losses, as more of Arminda's patients had died than were alive: "We are used to seeing them greet us, having conversations, looking for a way forward together. That makes us proud of work done well. But when a patient dies, we feel it." Volunteers often took setbacks per-sonally and suffered through feelings of guilt and sleepless nights. One of Arminda's colleagues told me: "I get this nervousness, a kind of stress, and loneliness, because there is often nothing more I can do." Arminda's comment, "I'm a person too," is a reminder that the volunteers were in situations of chronic uncertainty just like their patients and were often HIV positive themselves or caring for family members with AIDS.[28]

"WE CAN'T FIND THIS SPIRIT OF HELP"

Arminda had hoped her certifications and experience would translate into steady employment: "When we were trained, we were told we would be needed one day [as salaried workers]. Well, that day has not come." The recommended monthly incentive was usually half the amount Arminda made through her market stall, a significant sum despite being set below minimum wage, yet it was inconsistently provided and only for a relatively brief period of her career as a volunteer. Arminda expressed her frustration:

> We are expected to carry the burden of labor but not the benefits? Our organization has built a nice office. But those of us who do the work in the neighborhoods, this is not our office, and that hurts. We built that office, we built the organization. We arrive at the homes of the sick, and they say, "Mufudzi is here." We are Mufudzi. But we [volunteers] are the last to receive and the first to lose. Perhaps we should discuss selling the office.

The "work in the neighborhoods" was relating to and accompanying patients and their families. Arminda maintained it was unfair that the organization's administration materially benefited from her work while her aspirations for greater security went unfulfilled. It was not just insufficient remuneration that bothered Arminda, however, as much as the sense that she and her colleagues had been used and abandoned in the scale-up.

Arminda recalled her initial vision for the project, of a collective effort for self and communal improvement, with disappointment. She herself could be counted a success story: as a volunteer she enrolled in night school and became literate enough to compile the data and the monthly summary report for the group of volunteers she managed. But she noted her story was exceptional. We had just visited another volunteer that had suffered a stroke resulting in partial paralysis. Arminda reflected on the irony that this long-time volunteer was now worse off than the patients she had cared for. Her affliction was not amenable to ARVs and therefore did not qualify for the services for which they recruited. She was left with few protections despite her many years of service: "*Mamá* is sick, her arm is paralyzed, she can't work, what will she eat?" Arminda lamented. "A person who was working, today she has stopped, and what benefits does she have?" The organization had not been built on a foundation more sustainable than fickle donor support: "If we had better organized, we could have had a fund; we could help our volunteers like *Mamá* here. She is a single mother. What will she and her family eat?" She reflected on the prosocial spirit of the volunteers and mourned the absence of this spirit in other quarters:

> I think of that association in Zimbabwe. We started it alone, made our own contributions. We would all go sow seeds in someone's *machamba* today, tomorrow in someone else's. We built our houses together as well. We made the bricks, got the wood. Men cut. Women collected. It wasn't easy, but there was this spirit of help, support. Here in the city, we can't find this spirit of help.

While CHBC began as a grassroots effort based on solidarity, service, and sacrifice, the influx of resources and shifts in values introduced by the scale-up contributed to the fracturing of the organization and the collective identity of the volunteers. This loss of solidarity that Arminda experienced on a personal level with Mufudzi resonates with the larger transformations in the politics of governance and aid contributing to growing inequality in Mozambique.[29] Arminda drew a parallel between the feeling of being exploited by Mufudzi and foreign organizations and the history of the slave trade and forced labor in Mozambique, implying that these unequal and violently extractive dynamics persisted in the AIDS economy:

> There are many volunteers, and since they started they've been given what? Soap, T-shirts? Finally, we were given something from the coffers, money that came from other countries. But now, that well is empty. They [Mufudzi] have fallen on hard times. They depended on foreign countries. Why don't we have our own funds for our volunteers? . . . We know how to help one another, and we have our patients who rely on us . . . but who wants to work for nothing? They say that as we are black we are slaves of foreign countries. And not just this country, there are many countries in this situation.

Despite her frustration, Arminda maintained that she and her fellow volunteers would continue following their patients: "Those of us with this spirit, we still visit the sick." And she noted, "You can't just call this work. . . . [T]his isn't an enterprise or a business. It's more like a church. . . . This spirit doesn't appear for everyone." Arminda thought of their collectivity as animated by a spiritual vocation, as did most volunteers. But she also noted a double standard: "We've got this situation amongst the volunteers. We are dying and being buried in disgrace. We lack transportation, we lack coffins, nothing to cover even ourselves. Where is Mufudzi? . . . Why don't we have our own funds for our volunteers?" While the volunteers selflessly served their patients, they could not expect the same from their organization.

This may reflect the difficult reality of community-based organizations whose fortunes are tied to two- and five-year grant cycles. As Arminda bemoaned, "What are we to do, wait five more years to refill this empty well?" In some ways Mufudzi itself suffered from a lack of care, as the organization became collateral damage when its international funding dried up. However, neither the burden of labor nor the chronic uncertainties that the volunteers faced were equally shared. The volunteers were excluded from the program they had helped create.

EMPOWERMENT OR EXPLOITATION?

The intersection of the AIDS epidemic with a lack of infrastructure was a defining challenge to the AIDS treatment scale-up in
sub-Saharan Africa and contributed to the pandemic's catastrophic
toll.[30] In the absence of a functioning public health system, voluntary labor was a central feature of AIDS treatment interventions.[31]
CHBC volunteers are an incarnation of community health workers
(CHWs), global health actors often seen as a "homogenous and
unchanging 'resource' in the provision of health care."[32] In the Alma
Ata Declaration of 1978, the WHO identified CHWs as community
advocates for social change and one of the cornerstones of comprehensive primary health care.[33] Following this model, newly independent Mozambique's comprehensive national health system was
fronted by a cadre of CHWs called Agentes Polivalentes Elementares (APEs) and made impressive population health improvements
in a brief period.

With the economic crisis of the 1970s leading to structural adjustment in the 1980s, the Alma Alta vision of comprehensive primary
health care was replaced by a more technocratic approach emphasizing cost-effectiveness and targeted interventions. With the onset of
the civil war and the downsizing of the public health sector through
structural adjustment, Mozambique's APE program was not adequately supported on a national level and shrank or disappeared
in many regions. Contrary to the vision of the CHWs as agents of
social change espoused in the Alma Ata Declaration, CHBC volunteers were viewed more as technical fixes, low-cost patches on fragmented health-care systems. As the treatment scale-up proceeded,
CHBC volunteer networks, which began as disparate and desperate
local action in the face of overwhelming need, were absorbed by the
Integrated Health Networks.

The religious orientation of the volunteers was exploited by
Mufudzi, who claimed altruistic work should not be paid work. At
the same time, it rendered the volunteers suspect to donors, MISAU,

and NGOs, who were concerned that "all they do is pray." As the scale-up gained momentum, CHBCs became incorporated into a transnational effort funded and directed by donors. Community labor was seen as a stand-in and a stopgap for what was constructed as truly effective clinical care. This devalued both the nonbiomedical skills of CHBC and the people who were seen to embody and represent them: older, poorly educated women. Problems deemed "social," such as hunger and livelihood, were further marginalized. The ownership of the intervention was wrested from the hands of those who began it as the lifesaving technologies of HIV testing and ARVs became available.

The scale-up extracted volunteer labor from an available pool of cheap labor to initiate the expansion of HIV services. Over the course of the scale-up, while many individuals were partially employed, only a very small percentage converted this into long-term or formal employment. Many longtime volunteers, while acknowledging the ways they derived benefits from their labor, ultimately felt exploited and abandoned by the organizations that they themselves had helped create. Anthropologist James Ferguson argues such practices are part of a contemporary mode of governance he terms "neoliberal extraction" that divides Africa into a patchwork of secured, cared-for, usable "enclaves" and unusable, abandoned terrain.[34] This dynamic can be seen to operate within global health interventions, and here operates within the AIDS economy.[35] AIDS treatment interventions created clinical enclaves for the distribution of ARVs that depended on the extraction of volunteer labor from the under- and unemployed members of the community.

Global health interventions that rely on voluntary labor can be seen to produce a neoliberal subjectivity in which the self is conceptualized as "a flexible bundle of skills that reflexively manages oneself as though the self was a business" (also discussed in chapter 2 as Foucault's neoliberal *homo economicus*, the "entrepreneur of himself").[36] Volunteering was a kind of "hope labor" in which exposure and experience could possibly lead to future employment.[37]

We might understand the motivations and aspirations of volunteers like Arminda by following Ferguson's later argument that in African contexts characterized by labor surplus, social personhood, and ethics of interdependence, individuals seek to position themselves as dependents of more powerful persons and institutions and to establish relationships of mutual obligation that he terms "declarations of dependence."[38] In addition to their certifications, volunteers earned a status and a set of dependents themselves. Volunteering is a connection to powerful institutions—NGOs and the state—which mediate opportunities for education and self-improvement. These institutions offer a form of recognition and belonging and the potential for security and care. Yet the opportunities that now emerge from the intersections of state, transnational, and nongovernmental actors, which characterize the space of the AIDS economy, are "uncertain, transient, and precarious."[39] In contexts like central Mozambique, development projects like the global AIDS treatment scale-up often raise expectations without fulfilling them, and the partnerships that produce them are often short-lived and unstable.

Arminda's story emphasizes the importance of going beyond the notion of the CHW as a resource—an undifferentiated pool of cheap labor to be exploited in the name of cost-effectiveness and sustainability and who can be counted on to implement global health directives—without bringing individual thought and biography to bear. Arminda and her colleagues derived multiple benefits from their labor and took pride in their work and their service. Yet they felt let down and abandoned by Mufudzi, MISAU, and the AIDS treatment effort. The volunteers were caught between not having sufficient technical expertise, from the perspective of MISAU and funders, and the need to preserve their altruistic motives, from the perspective of Mufudzi administrators. The Mufudzi volunteers were ultimately discarded, deemed no longer usable, and Mufudzi itself collapsed as the intervention was "taken to scale."

5 Being Seen in the Day Hospital

Prior to the availability of ARVs in the Day Hospital, the NHS was overwhelmed by cases of AIDS, for which no treatment existed. Mozambique's once exemplary health system had been damaged by the civil war and by the austerity measures mandated by structural adjustment programs.[1] Government spending on health care declined from a high of 11 percent of GDP in the late 1970s to only 2 percent in 1996.[2] Under these conditions, Fátima, an HIV positive nurse and one-time association leader in Chimoio, recalled a need to have specialized care for HIV/AIDS:

> We created the Day Hospital to give special attention to people with HIV. People were not getting good care in the regular hospitals. They kept coming back, not getting better, and the staff just gave up. They told people to stop coming back because there was nothing they could do!

Clinical care at the Day Hospital was delivered by NHS physicians, medical assistants (*técnicos de medicina*), and nurses.[3] Donors financed the distribution of ARVs free of charge, and a foreign NGO trained and employed a specialized staff devoted to the process of enrolling, supporting, and tracking patients: two social workers, two statisticians, and twelve peer adherence counselors (*agentes terapêuticos*) recruited from the membership of associations of people living with HIV/AIDS. This auxiliary staff was mobilized not only to educate and counsel patients but also to monitor adherence, to avoid what northern donors and aid administrators feared could otherwise turn into an "antiretroviral anarchy" of resistance to ARV medications.[4] These fears, redolent with racist, colonial assumptions regarding "uncivilized Africans," proved unfounded but were baked into the treatment protocols that, after years of delay, finally arrived in Africa.

The Day Hospital mobilized the *Vida Positiva* language of empowerment and self-esteem to reinforce adherence to a new treatment regime and a new lifestyle. Fátima, the nurse described in the introduction, congratulated patients for increases in their CD4 count: "Keep doing what you are doing. Great job! Keep taking your medications!" Decreases prompted inquiries into causes of the problem and reprimands: "Are you taking your pills? Are you drinking? Smoking? Having unprotected sex? Has your partner tested?" Missed appointments, poor nutrition, worsening health, and especially problems with adherence to medications were seen as individual failures.

The focus on adherence as an individual task obscured the considerable structural obstacles many faced. I chatted with patients as they waited in the bright, bustling foyer of the Day Hospital, a space haunted by the ravages of AIDS embodied by skeletal patients. Crowded from the moment it opened its doors in the morning at 7:30 to when the final patients went home in the early afternoon, the Day Hospital bore witness to lifesaving care as patients recognized those who had gained weight and vitality. But establishing the criteria for acceptance into the ARV program—based on patients' attainment of individual indicators that made them worthy of treatment—entailed long delays and bitter disappointment, as the Day Hospital proved to be part of an inequitable treatment system that made it difficult for those patients who were already more vulnerable—poorer, sicker, and more isolated—to sustain access to care and to start ARVs. The focus of AIDS treatment programs on biology, behavior, and treatment readiness served to individualize the structural obstacles most patients faced.

THE DAY HOSPITAL: EXCEPTIONAL CARE

The arrival of ARV treatment in Mozambique was accompanied by attempts to reframe AIDS as a chronic disease "like any other."[5] These arguments came from activists combating stigma and the popular notion that AIDS was a death sentence, as well as health professionals who wanted AIDS patients to be treated in hospitals like all other patients and administrators who wanted to routinize and integrate HIV care into existing programs. Yet the scale of the AIDS epidemic and the deadly toll it took on the young and the otherwise healthy drove arguments that HIV was an exceptional disease requiring an exceptional response and led to the dramatic increase in funding that enabled the global scale-up of ARV treatment.

The scale-up of interventions dedicated specifically to HIV/AIDS treatment became the subject of long-standing global debates about "vertical" versus "horizontal" programming. Vertical programming allocated the majority of funding to disease-specific projects. Horizontal programming represented more broad-based improvements in public health, such as preventive medicine, primary care, and health workforce development.[6] Critics of vertical programs argue they divert resources from the needs of the general health system—and the broader social concerns of the majority of patients—toward one specific disease, creating inequalities and imbalances within health systems. The Mozambican government, favoring a more horizontal approach, wanted the AIDS treatment scale-up to proceed through the NHS and was opposed to the creation of a parallel treatment system.[7] But PEPFAR, the biggest funder of AIDS treatment, was highly "verticalized" and narrowly focused on HIV services only, providing funds to private NGOs and charities and creating parallel medical supply, data collection, and management systems dedicated to HIV/AIDS.[8] The result was often tense public-private partnerships, implemented differently all over the country.[9]

Twenty-three AIDS-focused outpatient Day Hospitals were constructed in Mozambique as enclaves of quality, accessible care with adequate medication supply, staff, and data monitoring and collection beside the decaying primary health care infrastructure of the public health system.[10] Unique supportive services—nutritional supplementation, transportation subsidies, and psychosocial support and counseling—were all aspects of care in the initial model of the Day Hospital. It was the center of an integrated health network model linking primary care services for HIV-positive patients, including ARV treatment, with VCTs, CHBC networks, and associations of people living with HIV/AIDS.[11] Despite the emphasis on community linkages on paper, in practice the care was biomedically driven and focused on delivery of ARVs, an imbalance that became more pronounced as the scale-up proceeded. While some patients, particularly those with resources and social capital, would experience an exceptional level of care, for others Day Hospitals reinforced already existing inequities in care.

In Chimoio, the Day Hospital (see figure 15) was officially a part of the NHS and was on the campus of the provincial hospital, which occupied an entire block in the *cidade de cimento*. The Day Hospital's main room consisted of a large, central foyer, with reception at the entrance. The foyer was well lit by sunlight streaming through skylights and filled with benches on which patients and family members waited to be called into the various rooms encircling the foyer where physicians, nurses, and *técnicos de medicina* performed their clinical exams. CHBC volunteers might drop patients off or wait with them there. The rooms around the foyer consisted of an infirmary with beds for the sickest patients, a patient records archive where information was entered into a computer database, and a room

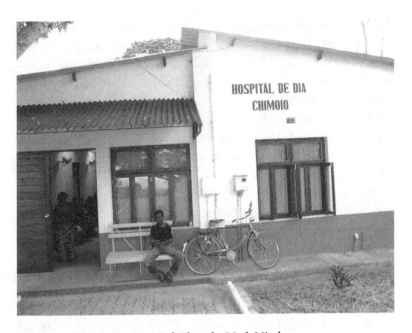

Figure 15. Chimoio Day Hospital. Photo by Mark Micek.

for staff meetings that doubled as an exam room. There were two nurses' offices, one for weighing and collecting vital signs, the other where nurse Fátima provided CD4 results to patients; two clinician exam rooms; a social worker's office; and a pharmacy, where ARVs and other medications were distributed. The walls featured colorful posters with characteristic HIV prevention slogans, such as "HIV/AIDS: Know More, Live More" and "Care for Yourself and Your Partner: Protect Yourselves from Sexually Transmitted Diseases." In the foyer, a television set played HIV education videos, some of them locally produced.

The process of being seen in the Day Hospital began with a positive test, either in the separate, stand-alone VCT center or in the main hospital. Patients who tested positive were given a small square of paper that served as their presumptive ticket into the Day Hospital and the broader AIDS economy. But this was only the first step toward receiving treatment and other potential benefits. Patients also had to navigate the crowded clinic and rigid protocols. One woman bringing her niece for a scheduled consult wanted to see if she, also registered at the Day Hospital as a patient, could be seen that day rather than return for her appointment the following week. She unsuccessfully pleaded, "Do you realize I spend 55 meticais (over 2 $US) for transport to each visit?" The receptionist apologized that the day's slots were all taken. Though transportation subsidies existed in theory, in practice they were difficult to obtain because of shifting criteria regarding eligibility of visits and availability of these funds. Many patients also complained that coming to the Day Hospital for anything meant losing an entire day.

Mornings in the clinic were overwhelming, with people standing, sitting, and milling around; names being called; doors opening and closing; and staff troubleshooting problems and shepherding patients, paperwork, and providers, all intermingled with smells of sweat, bleach, and dust or mud, depending on the weather. It was difficult to keep up with the social workers as they juggled their tasks as heads of support services. One veteran social worker, Pedro, would occasionally dab his brow with a handkerchief, allowing me to catch up as I followed him on his rounds. Short and wiry, Pedro articulated the challenges and uncertainty Day Hospital patients and staff faced:

> The patients here are often very sick, and they have received very little counseling regarding what they have and what it means. Beyond that, there are significant socioeconomic barriers to good care. We can subsidize the transportation costs of those who need to take a *chapa*, and there are limited food supplements from the World Food Program, but only once they are on treatment, not before. The majority receive no support; that is our reality.

While auxiliary supports such as food and transportation subsidies were unique, they were earmarked for those who managed to start ARVs. Other unique features of the Day Hospital were individual paper charts for each patient and statisticians employed to compile data—numbers of patients on ARVs, rates of adherence and dropout, rates of enrollment of men, women, and children—which donors required to monitor the treatment programs.[12] This emphasis on documentation and surveillance was an exceptional aspect of care in the Day Hospital as compared to the rest of the NHS, but it created additional burdens on health workers and patients, as care was often delayed due to missing documentation.

Social workers led a two-week training seminar for *agentes terapêuticos* on the basics of HIV/AIDS biology, counseling, and clinical care. Peer adherence counselors were recruited from associations of people living with HIV/AIDS, so they were local residents living with AIDS and often on ARVs themselves. They were close to the majority of patients in terms of lived experience, culture, language, and class and provided a link between the Day Hospital and local associations. These *agentes terapêuticos* had many formal duties, including counseling patients individually and in groups and conducting home visits to patients who had been lost to follow-up.[13] But they also managed many miscellaneous tasks in the Day Hospital required for daily operations—interpreting for clinicians who did not speak the local languages, reception, delivery of blood samples to the laboratory, mopping up vomit, and managing patient records, for example. In addition, they interfaced with the CHBC volunteers who brought their patients to the Day Hospital.

The Day Hospital was meant to be kept free of many of the constraints the NHS faced. While treatment in the NHS was ostensibly free, the civil war, bankruptcy, and structural adjustment had taken a toll on infrastructure, which forced user fees to be instituted. The Day Hospital had no user fees. Salaries of NHS public health workers were frozen by structural adjustment mandates, prompting a flight of professionals to the private and NGO sector. Pharmaceuticals were diverted to the black market (see figure 16), and patients had to purchase them in private pharmacies when stocks in public clinics ran out, a frequent occurrence outside the Day Hospital. ARVs and necessary antibiotics were available free of charge

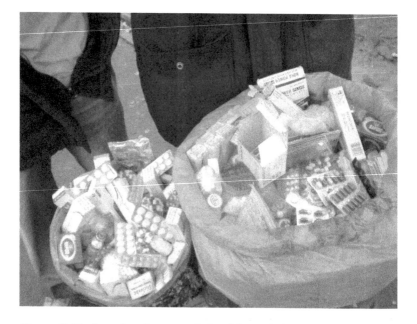

Figure 16. Black market pharmaceuticals sold in a Chimoio market.

in the Day Hospital, and the stocks were closely guarded. Unauthorized fees in the NHS increased as physicians, nurses, and other health-care workers struggled to feed their families on low public sector salaries.[14] NGO administrators worked to prevent assessment of under-the-table charges in the Day Hospital. When one *agente terapeûtico*—Oswaldo, hired from the Takashinga association—was caught asking for "special service" fees, he was swiftly dismissed by the NGO that paid his salary.

As ARV treatment scaled up, it was clearly experienced as something exceptional—special and specific to the AIDS crisis. This parallel system, however, focused narrowly on the scale-up of HIV services rather than the needs of the broader health system, creating inequities within the health system. With the emphasis on individual adherence and responsibility, Day Hospitals also compounded many of the preexisting challenges of the hollowed-out infrastructure, making people work to prove they deserved treatment. Even once ARVs existed in local clinics, there were considerable obstacles to accessing them, which led to inequities, hierarchies, and tensions.

EMPOWERMENT, RESPONSIBILITY, AND INDIVIDUALIZATION

There were two sets of criteria for initiation of ARVs, biological and social. New patients were assigned a number and had their blood drawn for laboratory analysis, including the CD4 cell count. If and when they met biological criteria, based on laboratory tests and HIV symptoms, the social worker would initiate the psychosocial evaluation to assess for the social criteria.[15] Social criteria were related to a patient's "psychological readiness" and ability to maintain adherence. Patients were educated about HIV/AIDS and ARVs and encouraged to live positively, practicing specific forms of self-care: to use a condom with every sexual encounter, to not ingest the herbal medicines of traditional healers, to maintain a good diet, to not physically overexert themselves, and to agree to a lifetime of adherence to antiretroviral medications. Patients beginning ARVs were asked to agree to these criteria.

The *Vida Positiva* booklet was handed out to new patients and circulated in associations prior to and during the early days of the treatment scale-up. The social workers' mission was to educate patients, preparing them for treatment by teaching them the importance of staying adherent and taking responsibility. Patients had to demonstrate a basic understanding of HIV infection and the AIDS illness, and whether they would be likely to maintain strict adherence to the twice-daily antiretroviral dosing. One patient, Florência, whose story was initially presented in chapter 3, had been thrown out of her family home by her in-laws because of her illness. She reflected on her treatment:

> When they give you those medications, they give you a little book. You
> read it, and if you decide to take it—because you are really going to
> take it—you have to take it for the rest of your life, no matter what. . . .
> It was difficult at first, sometimes I missed a dose, but now when it's
> time, I have my own internal signal. Missing is fatal.

While not every patient read the booklet or even had functional lit-
eracy in Portuguese, the social workers and *agentes terapêuticos*,
steeped in the discourse of living positively, introduced patients to
the principles of *Vida Positiva*: healthy living in body, mind, and
soul. Florência continued, "I need to increase my CD4, so I take my
medicines. I eat well. I try not to lose any sleep or have any vices."
Florência's disciplined self-care regimen resulted in improved
health, and she later successfully reconciled with her family.

The social workers assessed the social criteria for treatment
through a process of counseling and evaluation conducted over three
visits. The first and third visits were one-on-one counseling sessions
for the patient, while the second was a group counseling session.
In order to meet the social criteria, patients had to demonstrate a
basic understanding of HIV infection and the AIDS illness and the
need for strict treatment adherence as well as show they had sufficient social support to help them fill prescriptions even when ill
and unable to come to the pharmacy themselves. Social support was
formalized through the use of an adherence partner, a *testemunha*,
literally a "witness." Patients were asked to bring in a *testemunha*,
who was often a family member, who would learn, along with the
patient, the importance of adherence and positive living and could
assist the patient in maintaining these. Pedro explained, "If there's no
testemunha, then who can come to the hospital when they are sick?"
The *testemunha* was based on the "buddy system," developed in the
early days of the AIDS pandemic by North American groups like the
Gay Men's Health Crisis, of training volunteers to provide people suffering from AIDS emotional support and help with daily tasks.

This *testemunha* concept resonated with the language of the
Pentecostal churches. The notion of witnessing or testifying to the

presence of God in one's life is central to Pentecostal Christianity and also resonated with the AIDS testimonials in the associations, which bore witness to the lifesaving capacity of ARVs. In practice, however, at times this served as an additional barrier to the many patients who did not feel safe disclosing their diagnosis to family or friends. Some patients asked an *agente terapêutico* to serve as their *testemunha*, but with clinic enrollment increasing rapidly, this was not a viable alternative given the small number of adherence counselors and their ever-growing lists of duties. Patients and their family members were asked to take responsibility for being the first line of adherence support, standing in for the fragmented health system.

Patients who met the social criteria by demonstrating their understanding of the requirements, attending three counseling visits, and having a designated *testemunha* had their charts sent to the committee, which met weekly to approve all cases initiating ARVs. The first fourteen days of treatment were directly observed, which meant patients came to the clinic each morning to take their morning dose and then took their evening dose home with them.[16] At the clinic, a "TOD" room was designated for directly observed therapy (*tratamento observado direitamente*; TOD). TOD was required because the most severe side effects would occur during those initial days, but it also spoke to an anxiety about letting patients manage their treatment by themselves. Patients who lived too far away to make this practical or who were physically unable to return daily could take more medication with them and had a peer adherence counselor visit them. Pedro continued, "For those who do not earn 100 meticais [~US\$4] a month, this is difficult. But, if the patient can get here, we try hard to do what we can."

Pedro wearily listed the litany of obstacles there were to meeting criteria for treatment:

> Confidentiality and privacy in the family, for instance. We do not want to divulge results to the family unless the patient wants it. This can complicate the process. And then, of course, level of education. Many

people do not read or write, and this is a complicated treatment. And food? They must eat in order to recover.

Florência spoke directly to the hunger she experienced with ARV treatment: "The only thing I lack is food. If I'm hungry, even for two, three hours, I falter, I get dizzy, vertigo. The major problem is food, just food." Despite acknowledging these obstacles, Pedro did not question whether patients were capable of being adherent to treatment. He emphasized the importance of getting patients to understand these challenges and to agree to treatment despite them.

One morning in the Day Hospital, three patients who had asked Pedro for help with transportation costs gathered in his office. One of them had appealed to Pedro as "our father, our chief," positioning himself as a subordinate in a patron-client relationship. Pedro responded by lecturing the three patients about the need for responsibility, self-love, and a positive attitude:

> It is your responsibility to come in to the hospital. You are the ones who are sick and need care! How are you going to do this? What will happen when this program that gets you free treatment ends?. . . I am not giving life to anyone. You have to live, for yourself, for your responsibilities.

Pedro managed to be stern and still maintain a sense of humor and levity with his mini-lecture. He relied on the precepts of the *Vida Positiva* curriculum:

> You have ARVs. Don't you know that you can live for 20, 30, 40 more years? I always ask you, on each day that is born, think and say, "I love myself." Don't stay afflicted! It is you that must get through each week! We know that what we provide isn't enough, but they are the conditions that exist. You can't leave here sad.

Pedro advised the patients to practice self-love and to not remain sad, attempting to buttress their self-esteem, individual responsibility, and accountability. In the popularization of the psychoneuro-immunological paradigm of *Vida Positiva*, remaining sad, upset, or stressed out actually could stimulate the HIV virus, while being relaxed and carefree encouraged the virus to sleep and remain dormant. Pedro was thus providing advice for healthy living as well as orientation to being a compliant and adherent subject of HIV treatment. The patients did seem brightened up by his enthusiastic response, even as they were refused money for transport. This brief interaction illustrated the ways individuals were asked to compensate for inadequate infrastructure as well as the tension between the model of the responsible, self-sufficient neoliberal subject and pre-existing patron-client systems "hoping for help from a 'patron' with resources to distribute."[17] Pedro's encouragement to his patients to be autonomous contrasts with the legacy of social relations as characterized by dependence and redistribution, with superiors bearing responsibility to care for their dependents.[18] This seemed to be the assumption of the patients who approached Pedro. Pedro exhorted his patients to take responsibility for themselves, citing the overwhelming need and the limitations of the health-care system. This reflects the socialization of scarcity pervasive in contemporary public sector spaces: the assumption that there are limited resources for health, and that shortfalls and trade-offs are inevitable and unavoidable.[19] This contrasted with the ethos of *estamos juntos* that was popular in the early days of independence, when robust public programs were designed to meet social needs.[20]

Pedro also expressed his concerns about the health system's ability to sustain the treatment program: "We have adequate treatment for now, but how long will it be for free? How long will the donors stay?" He did not have faith in the threadbare public health infrastructure or that the donor benevolence that provided free ARVs would be indefinite. He was familiar with the mercurial history of development trends that gave most interventions short lives and fostered the perpetual sense of scarcity. Pedro had seen projects and priorities come and go in the transitions of the previous decades, and he did not feel he could make any guarantees regarding what future structures might be in place to support ARV treatment.

TRIAGE, EXCLUSION, AND ABANDONMENT

Patients struggled to meet the demands of the enrollment process. Nilza, a thin woman with a weathered look whom I met in the Day Hospital waiting area wearing a *capulana* headscarf and wrap, had been declared ready to start ARVs in August, but she had no one at home to serve as her *testemunha*, she was too sick and frail to come every day, and no *agente terapêutico* lived near her. She disappeared until four months later, when she returned accompanied by a niece. She had diarrhea, however, that she needed to resolve before starting ARVs, so she received a prescription for antibiotics and lined up at the pharmacy, further prolonging the initiation of ARV treatment. Julia, a young woman Elena had recruited for treatment, frequently missed appointments in order to avoid disclosing her HIV-positive status to her mother-in-law. Numerous roadblocks within the health system delayed treatment as well: blood samples that sat out for too long and needed to be redrawn, thus necessitating yet another appointment; broken equipment; no physicians being present on appointment dates; lost charts; and misplaced paperwork.

Just showing up at the Day Hospital for care was perceived as risky for many who feared revealing their positive status to others. Privileged patients who were known to staff could avoid this kind of scrutiny by arranging to be seen in private and bypassing many of the lines, the group counseling, and the TOD process. Some patients who could afford the cost and time went to Day Hospitals outside of their home areas to try to avoid being seen by people they knew. A schoolteacher arranged to discreetly receive her medications at a bench on the hospital grounds. Employees of the NHS and the NGO providing technical assistance bypassed the crowded, time-consuming, and highly visible routes to treatment by disguising their clinical visits as professional meetings or by arranging them after hours. Public employees questioned whether they should apply for the disability benefit their positive serostatus made them eligible for because the application "passes through many sets of hands, all the way to the governor," as one social worker warned her patient. They feared losing their jobs if their serostatus was revealed, despite official legal protections.

An internal review in October 2005 found the average time between initial identification as ARV eligible according to biological criteria and first day of treatment was three months, but noted that some cases took as long as a year. Between January 2004 and June 2005, 50 percent of the adult patients eligible for ARVs did not receive them. The majority of these patients who were eligible for treatment but had not started died while awaiting treatment. The lengthy and elaborate period of evaluation preceding treatment, combined with health system inefficiencies, served as a de facto triage system that excluded the sickest and those who had difficulties making repeated visits. This system may have ensured high adherence rates in the clinic, but at the cost of treatment delays associated with a high mortality rate.

THE FACTS OF POSITIVE LIFE

Once they met the biological criteria, patients began the group counseling session that preceded treatment initiation. These sessions reinforced the new concepts and responsibilities patients were being taught. Central to the counseling was the focus on individual responsibility and the need to make treatment initiation a conscious choice and commitment. One of the social workers at the Day Hospital, Adélia, asked for an affirmative embrace of treatment and emphasized the daily obligations it demanded. "You have more time to consider this treatment, if you want it or no."

In these sessions, patients were introduced to the concept of the CD4 count. Day Hospital staff used it as an indicator of proper lifestyle. The CD4 count was understood to decrease with bad behaviors such as unprotected sex, taking traditional medications, and alcohol and tobacco use, and to increase with healthy behaviors, such as taking ARVs and sleeping and eating well. Adélia gave everyone a sticky note with their CD4 count written on it and asked each person to read their number in turn:

> Don't forget these numbers. Any person who is alive has this number. It is the number of defenders we have in our bodies, the soldiers that protect us so we don't get sick. 1,000, 2,000 and up, that's a healthy person.

Adélia reinforced the new concepts of CD4 counts and immune systems, "When these numbers go down, that's when diseases, diarrhea, cough, fever, enter. That's why you are sick. The virus eats our bodies from the inside." She individualized the virus, cloaked in the unique uniform of particular bodies: "Each body is unique and has a different virus, dressed in the uniform of your body."

The demands of living positively were read into the CD4 count. In her individual sessions with patients, Fátima also used the CD4 count as a kind of moral barometer, an objective measure of appropriate self-care, a technology of visibility that seemed to make an individual's intimate habits available for clinical scrutiny.[21]

Counseling at the Day Hospital was saturated with the moralism of *Vida Positiva*, the associations, and churches. Adélia Christianized ARVs, calling them a cross to bear, "This medicine, it is a cross. It is not a good thing. We do not wish for it. But it is a burden we must bear, twice a day, every day." In one session, Adélia gave examples of the ways individuals go astray, through drinking and unprotected sex, reinforcing this moralism:

> There are people who drink while they are taking medications, who have unprotected sex. It is not my health that is harmed. Each person cares for himself. . . . Some say since we are positive we can have sex

without a condom. But this isn't so. . . . You will re-infect each other and create resistance. Your CD4 won't go up even when you take these medications. The medications will become useless. For that reason, from now on, whenever we have sex, it is with a condom.

The focus on CD4 count took root and branched out past the walls of the clinic, where people compared CD4 counts and speculated about the causes of increases or decreases, since CD4 counts were retaken every six months. An activist explained: "You can't have vices. When you take care of yourself, CD4 increases. If it is not increasing and you are on treatment, you are doing something wrong." When word got out that the count of one association member rose above 1,000, he was heartily congratulated. When someone else's CD4 count was rumored to have decreased, speculation abounded: "Ah, it's that husband of hers, he won't use condoms. You see what happens!" or "I told you, he's a heavy drinker."

The CD4 count was yet another way the illness was individualized and moralized, and health was tied to individual choice and behavior. An explanation for a decline in CD4 count was always sought in a patient's habits and choices. Anthropologist Johanna Crane notes the concept of resistance had a moral framing as "a form of negative payback for poor adherence."[22] One feared reason CD4 count might not rise was infection with a virus that had developed resistance to the generic, first-line ARVs. While higher rates of adherence are commonly believed to guard against resistance, some degree of resistance will inevitably develop in a setting of widespread treatment. In fact, ARV drug resistance has been found to vary by antiretroviral therapeutic class and is just as likely to be found among the most highly adherent patients as among those with poor adherence.[23] Second-line antiretroviral medications, to be used when the first line failed due to the development of resistance, were not available as generics and were thus expensive and difficult to access in Mozambique. Resistance was thus not completely tied to an individual's ability to be adherent but could also be understood as a trait of the specific ARV type and the result of drug pricing. Despite this fact, patients were usually blamed when their CD4 counts did not rise.

This moralism was clearest when sex and fertility were discussed. Pedro expressed concerns about sexual behavior, reinfection, and the potential development of ARV-resistant virus. This reflected fears that resistance could result from poor adherence to ARVs or from reinfection, which occurred when an already HIV positive individual was infected with a new strain of HIV from another infected individual:

> We are very concerned about resistance. Are we causing more problems by starting treatment? We have to educate them. This isn't an aspirin! It's a serious treatment, with serious risks, and for life! And if they do not understand the consequences of unprotected sex and reinfection? Just today, I spoke to a patient who has been here, getting care for over a year, and his wife is pregnant! How could he?

Pedro saw unprotected sex and pregnancy in the setting of HIV infection as a violation of the terms of ARV treatment and considered withdrawing treatment from these unruly subjects. Unprotected sex was seen as immoral behavior that would then result in antiretroviral resistance.

An assumption of *Vida Positiva* in the clinic was that AIDS patients would no longer reproduce. When someone who was HIV positive became pregnant, they were reprimanded and blamed for spreading the virus and for causing resistance. Pedro explained:

> They are re-infecting each other! We've had discussions of how to handle these cases—should we stop treating those who get pregnant? So far, we haven't. I used to get really upset about these kinds of patients, but I can't anymore, I would just drive myself crazy. In five years, I worry [these ARVs] will be obsolete [due to resistance].

This individualized the epidemic itself, despite the existence of clear structural drivers of the epidemic, such as poverty and inequality.[24] It also served to further isolate people with AIDS, especially women, from their social networks, as child bearing was a key marker of social status and adult competence, and a way to secure social support. I found this particularly puzzling, because as a medical student, I had been involved in births of HIV negative children to HIV positive mothers on ARVs in the United States. This option was not sanctioned for Mozambican patients during the initial stages of treatment scale-up, even while women taking ARVs were in fact giving birth to HIV negative children. They were asked to sacrifice their vital social connections and to bear the responsibility for halting the epidemic through their individual behaviors. It seemed to be yet another form of structural violence imposed on Mozambicans living with HIV/AIDS.

In contrast to the "kinds of patients" Pedro was concerned about, a select few did manage to adhere to the principles of *Vida Positiva* and gain wider access to the benefits to be found within the AIDS economy. Florência's adherence to ARV treatment, for example, had helped her receive food supplements from the Day Hospital, and after she had regained her health and her life, she was able to reconcile and reshape her relationship with her family. Florência was also eventually hired to work as an *agente terapêutico* in a Day Hospital. She internalized a strong, conscious choice to commit to ARVs and her adherence to ARVs as a part of her being—"I have my own internal signal"—and tried to live morally, free of vices. And yet even the model patient went hungry prior to her obtaining regular employment as a peer adherence counselor. As Adélia told patients in the counseling sessions, "You've got to eat; otherwise how will you get better? Eat a little, relax. Eat a little, rest. This medication is strong! If you don't eat, you'll feel bad, and you won't get better." This was easier said than done for most patients, and persistent hunger was commonly pointed to and seemed to stand for the shortcomings of the treatment programs.

WORTHY OF TREATMENT

When ARVs were first developed in the global north, the argument that Africans were "unsanitary subjects ... incapable of adopting

[a] modern medical relationship to the body, hygiene, illness, and healing," was used to justify withholding treatment from millions of people in Africa.[25] This racist and classist assumption regarding the ability of Africans to adhere to treatment was structured into treatment programs, as Mozambicans had to earn access to ARVs by meeting not only clinical criteria but the social criteria that ensured they could be "sanitary citizens ... credited with understanding modern medical concepts and behaving in ways that make them less susceptible to disease."[26] Even once ARVs existed in local clinics in central Mozambique, there were considerable obstacles to accessing them, with inevitable delays caused by lost blood samples and broken machinery, and the time-consuming process of earning eligibility. Most poor patients were viewed with suspicion, and the protocols assumed most were constitutionally incapable of maintaining adherence to ARVs and living positively. Cases like Florência's were seen as the exceptions that proved the rule. Yet it was structural factors, not individual faults, that most often interfered with treatment access and adherence.[27]

The imposition of social criteria was structured by fears, such as those Pedro expressed, that poor adherence would result in resistant strains of HIV, rendering the cheap, generic medications being administered as first-line treatment obsolete. These fears that Africans were incapable of maintaining a high level of adherence justified delays in the introduction of ARVs to the continent. A series of projects across the global south that demonstrated that patients were capable of high adherence rates despite living in abject poverty finally changed this perception.[28] Crane points out a dark implication of this triumph that paved the way for the global scale-up of AIDS treatment:

> While this rehabilitation of the African patient was a boon in the fight for global treatment access, it came at the cost of providing discriminatory health policies and practices with scientific legitimacy. By allowing drug resistance to continue to be framed as the outcome of individual failure, this positive re-imagining of the African patient

reinforced the same bitter logic as its negative predecessor: that some people merited treatment, and others did not.[29]

Even as treatment would become available in Mozambique, free of charge through the NHS, the notion persisted that ARVs needed to be protected from the development of resistance and that people had to prove themselves capable of adherence and worthy of treatment. In a provider meeting, the Day Hospital clinical chief called for 100 percent adherence rates: "Soon we will have many more patients on ARVs, and it will get more difficult to follow them. Resistance is our priority. We need to account for everyone who begins treatment. Otherwise it will look ugly." The priority was ensuring high rates of adherence first, before expanding access to treatment. The "ugliness" in the clinical chief's comment referred to the specter of widespread resistance.

Suzana, whom I had initially met at a workshop sponsored by the association of which Fátima was president, worked with Fátima in the Day Hospital as an *agente terapêutico*. Suzana identified those who were HIV positive but were not accessing treatment as "people who think ARVs cause disease." If treatment was available free of charge to all who met the criteria, then those who were not receiving treatment must be making a choice not to or must not believe that the treatment is effective. They therefore did not deserve treatment. This was the dark side of the discourse of individual responsibility.

The result was the creation of the social criteria for treatment, construed as a kind of *moral criteria*, that functioned as additional barriers to the poorer, sicker, and more precarious patients who were likely to have more difficulty with treatment due to the many obstacles they faced. The social criteria compounded those obstacles, maintaining an evaluation process that effectively eliminated 50 percent of the sickest and most precarious patients. Though these criteria resulted in fewer patients being treated overall, they did contribute to selecting those who had a higher likelihood of adherence and thus had a higher likelihood of successful treatment. Fears of

resistance stalled initial efforts to provide ARVs in Africa and continued to create obstacles to treatment access even within the treatment programs.

Access to ARVs was shaped by inequality and colonial legacies
on both global and local levels. Just as in the associations and the
CHBC networks, the language of *Vida Positiva* and the attitudes of
providers in the Day Hospital were infused with the ideas of "civilization," "enlightenment," and "modernity." That language contrasted
the figure of the ideal self-reflexive, independent, responsible, and
obedient patient with the ignorant, backward, superstitious, and
African patient. The seemingly objective criteria for treatment relied
on precepts that mapped onto the colonial dualism of civilization
and tradition of the Indigenato. While the policies of the Indigenato
were no longer in effect, its social and cultural legacy was alive.
Though the majority of physicians and nurses were Mozambican,
they tended to be of a higher social class than most patients and
often didn't speak any of the indigenous languages that were part
of the multilingual Chimoian landscape. Overt signs of cultural and
class difference were singled out for derision. This resulted in poor
treatment of patients who were seen to embody the characteristics
of "African tradition," through dress or language.[30]

One physician who noticed a colored thread a young female
patient wore around her wrist asked the patient: "What is this?"
Looking down and smiling sheepishly, she answered, "Nothing."
The doctor mocked, "Is it grandma?," alluding to the veneration
of ancestral spirits. Wearing colored string is a practice in many
AICs meant to provide spiritual protection to vulnerable people,
especially those who are ill. As mentioned in chapter 3, association
member Amílcar had also surreptitiously shown me his as he
waited in the Day Hospital. The gulf in class and culture between
physician and patient was visible in the distinction between the
woman's *capulana* on her slight frame and the red thread she wore
and the sporty sunglasses perched on top of the physician's head.
The physician wore a cell phone on a lanyard around his thick

neck, which he faithfully answered whenever it rang even while seeing patients.

When these clinicians saw signs of class and cultural difference— *capulanas*, colored string, and wasted bodies—they also saw ignorance, which led them to blame their patients for their misfortune, exaggerating their agency and blaming the victims of structural violence.[31] Challenges caused by deficiencies in the health system and the blind spots of the intervention itself were attributed to patients. A two-month-old baby who had not gained weight since the first week of life was brought in by the grandmother because the mother was sick at home. The doctor chided the grandmother, grumbling, "This child is hungry, not sick." When the physician saw another malnourished infant with the mother, the father was brought in from the waiting area and was asked why he was not buying formula for his child who was not gaining weight. He told the doctor that he had no work so could not afford it. The physician later told me that he did work, but "he wants the hospital to do everything for them." To another mother who similarly said she did not have money for formula, the physician scolded: "Come now, you don't even have money to buy these little necessities you need?" This physician responded to malnutrition and hunger in children as evidence of parental neglect and irresponsibility.

After a patient reported being tired, one physician replied: "If you were rich, you could pay someone to do your housework, to do your shopping, cleaning. But, since you are not, you've got to work hard to survive." To another patient asking when she would be seen, a nurse tersely replied, "Look, you are the one who is sick." When a patient asked whether a medication she had been given was causing a specific side effect, the nurse responded "only in your head!"

In such cases, hospital staff seemed to be taking out their frustrations with the challenging circumstances on the patients themselves. They practiced in a system in which pharmacies often lacked medication and patients lacked the means to buy many basic necessities, laboratory tests were routinely delayed or nonexistent, and their services were in high demand but they lacked the proper tools and supports to successfully practice the kind of medicine they were trained in. One health worker who had worked during the revolution recalled, "We thought we were building something then. Now, morale is quite low." Morale was kept low by structural adjustment mandates that froze health sector salaries and continued to starve the NHS. This period of the scale-up may have been a particularly frustrating time for clinicians. Initial pilot projects hired clinicians as consultants on lucrative, short-term contracts, but these incentives disappeared when treatment was offered by the NHS, undermining the physicians' willingness to work in the Day Hospital. A fee-for-service private clinic opened in Chimoio in the mid-1990s, and during my fieldwork a new private hospital was being built. Many physicians and nurses in Mozambique maintained both public and private practices and often focused on the latter at the expense of the former. I observed private-pay patients who were not HIV positive nonetheless come to the Day Hospital for consultations with physicians.

ARV TREATMENT AND FOOD DISTRIBUTION: "THIS IS A DIFFERENT DISEASE!"

Patients in the Day Hospital frequently asked staff about receiving food aid. A young female patient asked Adélia, "Isn't there food for patients here?" Adélia responded curtly, "Do you go to clinics expecting to be fed?" The patient responded, "No, but this is a different disease," to which Adélia responded, "No it isn't. How do you know what disease different patients have?" The patient recounted the story of how she had gone to get water from her neighborhood's pump and been yelled at by other women who said, "You lost your baby to this disease. You will contaminate us! You are spoiled. You cannot be here." She asserted that the illness was different, that it resulted in social exclusion and made it difficult to attend to her daily needs.

She tried her best to be seen and heard in the Day Hospital, in the hopes of receiving the support she knew existed. Adélia shook her head, and repeated to her something she had told me many times before: "Food is not treatment. Food is a support that some receive for some time, but it ends. Food is not treatment."

The Day Hospital had 250 food baskets to distribute among people on ARVs. It was the job of the social workers and adherence counselors to decide who was to receive this food for three months, the initial phase of treatment when side effects were likely to be the most severe. They met every two weeks to discuss who would be assigned available baskets. In between meetings, peer adherence counselors were to visit the patients who were beginning ARVs in order to see who was most in need: those who did not work, who had multiple dependents, and who lived in the most "vulnerable" situations. At the meeting, they presented the cases of the most deserving. Others would ask questions or offer information they knew regarding the patient's situation. Five to ten percent of the cases I heard were deemed ineligible, often because a patient was suspected of working or feigning "vulnerability." When the case of one patient who presented herself as a single mother was brought up, an activist insisted she had a male partner whom she hid from the health staff. Patients like this, who showed too much agency to be considered victims, were passed over. Patients deemed eligible were put on a list to replace those whose three months of eligibility had ended. As the number of patients grew, however, it became more difficult for the twelve *agentes terapêuticos* to visit them all.

Patients whose three months had expired frequently made appeals to social workers for extensions because their economic situations had not improved. The staff acknowledged that the demand exceeded the available baskets. Yet even as the number of patients on ARVs doubled, from 873 in September 2005 to 1,660 in July 2006, the number of food baskets that were available through the clinic remained the same, 250. Inevitably, each decision regarding who would receive one turned someone else away. Social workers and peer adherence counselors bore the brunt of the pleas of patients who felt wrongfully excluded, but protested there was little they could do. By 2010, food was meant to be provided according to strict biometric criteria, such as body mass index less than 18, but these criteria were not always adhered to.

Nearly half of Mozambicans suffer from chronic malnutrition.[32] Malnutrition is linked with increased susceptibility to HIV infection, and food insecurity has been found to contribute to the spread of HIV, to correlate with worse adherence to ARVs, and to impede recovery.[33] Despite the centrality of food and nutrition in susceptibility to HIV and overall well-being, most administrators I spoke to linked the provision of food with two explicit medical goals: to improve treatment adherence and overall health outcomes. Thus, hunger was reduced to an obstacle to care and recovery rather than acknowledged as a key factor in the epidemic. Administrators of the pre-scale-up pilot treatment programs outside of the NHS recalled that clinic attendance improved dramatically when food was provided to patients and their entire families. As the NHS treatment program grew in size and numbers of patients, the amount of food did not keep pace with the number of people enrolling in treatment. It never was scaled up nationally alongside ARVs.

When Florência had used up her eligibility for food supplements from the Day Hospital, she was occasionally able to get food from a local Catholic mission. She looked for work as a domestic servant, but she felt that her HIV status, which was publicly known because she "broke the silence" on World AIDS Day, made her less employable—a stigma also suffered by Adélia's patient as she tried to get water. But Florência, who lived with her nine-year-old daughter and four-year-old son, who was also on ARVs, ultimately was able to access important resources on the basis of her diagnosis. In addition to lifesaving antiretrovirals, she received the more elusive benefit of the AIDS economy, employment in the Day Hospital as an *agente terapêutico*.

REINFORCING INEQUALITIES

Global access to AIDS treatment has always been structured by inequality. Prior to the global scale-up, northern donors and aid administrators feared the twin challenges of inadequate infrastructure and poorly educated patients rendered AIDS treatment in Africa unsustainable—that is, too costly to be feasible. In the words of USAID head Andrew Natsios, patients in Africa would not maintain strict adherence because they "do not know what watches and clocks are. They do not use Western means of telling time."[34] Despite the fears of resistance, the ARVs that were eventually made available in Africa were the cheapest and the type most likely to be susceptible to the development of resistance.[35] Economic considerations trumped public health concerns.

When ARVs were scaled-up in Mozambique, unequal access to treatment persisted, even within the Day Hospitals providing the medications. Patients and providers had to contend with a poorly funded and hollowed out infrastructure and with the principal donor, PEPFAR, channeling its considerable resources outside the public sector and the NHS and toward foreign NGOs. The emphasis placed on adherence rates and the fear of ARV resistance added additional pressure on a threadbare and stressed health system and on precarious patients struggling to survive. ARVs were available to those who were able to prove themselves worthy of treatment by fulfilling not just the biological criteria, but also the social criteria for treatment, which were consonant with the precepts of living positively. The solution for those working on the front lines in the Day Hospital, like Pedro, Adélia, Fátima, and the peer adherence counselors, was to counsel and teach their patients and their peers to be responsible and self-sufficient, drawing from the *Vida Positiva* techniques for self-care and management.

Writing about social welfare reform in the United States in the early 1980s, sociologist Barbara Cruikshank argues that such "technologies of subjectivity" promise to resolve social problems by encouraging individuals to look within themselves and recognize their "individual personal and social responsibility [for self-care]" as part of "a social movement premised upon the limits of politics and the welfare state, the failures of . . . democracy and upon the inability of government to control conflict."[36] These "technologies of subjectivity" were imposed on treatment in Mozambique in the context of structural adjustment austerity measures that decimated social welfare programs. In order to earn ARVs, one had to be a subject who lived positively—that is, who understood one's illness and the need for treatment in biomedical terms; was responsible for oneself; practiced specific forms of self-care; and was future-oriented, resourceful, and obedient. This subjectivity was connected to a form of transnational governmentality that circulated and established the mechanisms of neoliberal governance.[37] It also resonated with evangelical theology, based on individual grace and accountability.[38] Even those who would gain access to ARVs, however, often found themselves hungry.

In order to earn access to ARVs, patients in Mozambique had to prove themselves worthy of treatment by fulfilling not just the biological criteria but a set of social criteria for treatment that were consonant with the precepts of living positively, which itself was linked to the pernicious colonial dualism distinguishing Western modernity from African tradition and relegating the African to the realm of ignorance. These concerns were justified by fears of drug resistance that would make "the developing world a veritable 'petri dish' for new, treatment-resistant HIV strains," strains that an editorial in the medical journal *The Lancet* warned might "boomerang back to the West."[39] As Crane pointed out, the main obstacle to treatment was framed as Africa itself—"its weak governments, lack of trained physicians, poor laboratory facilities, impoverished and malnourished patients, and 'dirty water and mud roads."[40] Yet rather than rebuilding this infrastructure, the treatment interventions focused on shaping those who received treatment into forward-looking, modern neoliberal subjects living positively and ignored, minimized, or individualized the structural obstacles. Only the patients embodying this subject position were granted access to ARVs.

The "AIDS exceptionalism," much discussed throughout the African continent, resulted in inequities on multiple scales, internal and external to health systems, including an internal brain drain of professionals to AIDS programs and fewer resources for other health and social problems.[41] The acknowledgment of these challenges led to the shift to integration of HIV testing and ARV into primary health care services in Mozambique, a process that was implemented toward the end of my research. This mainstreaming of ARV treatment was justifiable from a health services perspective, as it would bring the resources earmarked for AIDS into the NHS and ideally strengthen the overall system rather than creating a parallel track for one disease.[42] Yet when this happened, many people living with AIDS who relied on the Day Hospital experienced this as an abandonment and responded with public demonstrations, often organized by associations.[43] Pedro's fears about the sustainability of the treatment programs seemed to be realized, as much of the adherence support infrastructure that existed—peer adherence counselors, food supplementation, specialized counseling, the *testemunha*—imperfect and limited as it was, would have its funding withdrawn when HIV/AIDS care ceased to function as a specialty service and Day Hospitals closed in favor of general primary care clinics.

6 Hunger as Embodied Critique

While Mozambicans told me stories of dramatic recoveries due to antiretrovirals, they were often embedded within complex narratives about the reality of living with ARVs. In a region with high rates of food insecurity, malnutrition, unemployment, and cyclical drought, hunger was a frequent topic of conversation. In her examination of hunger in Northeast Brazil, anthropologist Nancy Scheper-Hughes argues that "the biological, psychological, and symbolic meanings of hunger are merged in the experience of bodies that are mindful and minds that are culturally embodied."[1] Scheper-Hughes proposed a framework for understanding the body as "individually and collectively experienced, as socially represented in various symbolic and metaphorical idioms, and as subject to regulation, discipline, and control by larger political and economic processes."[2] This perspective approaches hunger as both a physiological sensation and a language rich in symbolic meaning that sheds light on the dynamics of social relations. It lends a more embodied and experiential resonance to the politically symbolic "politics of the belly" in Africa.[3]

These theoretical perspectives frame my understanding of hunger as a physiological sensation and also as an idiom for considering relations of care and dynamics of power.

The hunger that was experienced and discussed in the context of AIDS treatment communicated, directly and indirectly, important characteristics of the AIDS economy from the perspective of those navigating it. The comment "all I eat is ARVs" was a critique made by HIV positive Mozambicans who recognized the substantial investments in AIDS treatment, but felt the interventions ignored the conditions of poverty and hunger that made them vulnerable to illness in the first place. An intensified hunger emerged as a side effect of this treatment system, not only as a physiological consequence of the medication and a result of improved health (in a context of poverty and food insecurity), but also as an embodied critique of an exclusionary intervention whose benefits proved ultimately insufficient. That ARVs caused hunger is itself a potent representation of how the infusion of vast sums of donor money for AIDS treatment still left the Mozambican majority underfed, underemployed, and deeply impoverished due to ongoing neoliberal austerity measures. In this final chapter, I explore the hunger that was the outcome of AIDS treatment interventions and articulate calls for alternative ethics of interdependence and redistribution and for a politics of justice.

"NOT LIKE NORMAL HUNGER"

Elena, who had initially introduced me to the associations that had emerged in the AIDS scale-up and was working as an adherence counselor, an *agente terapêutico*, in the Day Hospital, agreed that the treatment seemed to provoke something unique:

> This hunger is different than a normal hunger. The hunger begins to really gnaw right here (putting her hand on her stomach). Sometimes at night, even after eating dinner, you sleep and around midnight,

one o'clock, it seems like you never ate, and you need to awake and eat at night. You can't sleep on that hunger.

Elena added that the hunger could be considered a sign of improvement:

> ARVs, yes, when a person takes them, they provoke hunger, and that [the return of an appetite, hunger] is a positive effect. That is to say that it is giving a good effect on the organism, because when you feel a lot of hunger, and you have food and eat well, the tendency is to fatten up.

Fattening up was a sign of improved strength and health, while losing weight indicated illness or struggle. The key, of course, was having food to assuage the hunger. In the absence of food, this hunger represented another problem in addition to AIDS. In the words of Batista, whom I met in Elena's association: "My body is well, but this hunger, it's another illness!" For those struggling to make ends meet, the hunger provoked by ARVs was frightening and was experienced, or at least referred to, as another illness.

Poor appetite is a common problem for people with HIV/AIDS. It can have multiple causes, including infections, pain (especially in the mouth or gut), depression, anxiety, or fatigue. Though the feeling of hunger may disappear, suppressed appetite leads to reduced nutritional intake, caloric deficiency, loss of muscle mass, and the characteristic wasting syndrome. ARVs effectively unmask the hunger of patients who had been previously starving to death without feeling it. ARVs may also contribute to hunger—even *cause* hunger, as was claimed—by increasing metabolism, which results in an increased need for caloric intake.[4] Yet there was more behind this talk of hunger than a physiological sensation. When people talked about a medication that made them hungry, they were using an embodied moral language to critique an incomplete and inadequate treatment. Patients were being told they should eat with their medications, but fewer and fewer were being given food. Indeed, they were given pills, but not food.

A woman with high, defined cheekbones and a fiery disposition, Mayita lived with her mother and three children and worked in the market. When I spoke with her about the comments of others related to hunger and ARV treatment, she agreed that she experienced a prodigious hunger in the beginning of her treatment, but she also recalled that at that time, "We did not have good conditions." Recently, her family had been able to cultivate their *machamba*, so she had not been experiencing hunger because she had enough food to eat. Others in precarious conditions complained more bitterly about this hunger. Victoria for example, commented, "Some nights I've suffered with hunger. When it starts, sometimes I end up going to the neighbors [to ask for food]." Josepha echoed, "When I go to sleep at 10, I'll wake up, *epa*, now the belly, it's got nothing, and it's even worse when the sun comes up if I haven't eaten by then." Others, like Madalena, were specific about the ARV-hunger connection: "This medicine, it bites. It is different, yes, not like normal hunger. If I don't eat when I take it, I tremble and shake. It is said this medicine will kill you if you don't eat with it." This idea that the medicine was so powerful it could kill was one I heard in the mid-2000s when ARVs first became available, as well as in 2010. This spoke to a much more threatening aspect of the hunger and was not necessarily a sign of a body in recovery.

Volunteers shared with me their impression that many people did not want to start ARVs because they caused hunger. Elena told me of patients she saw in the Day Hospital who stopped taking their medications because they did not have food to eat. She added that one such patient had recently visited her at home, saying, "I've gone days without [food]. I had to stop taking medicine on account of food. That medicine provokes hunger! These medications of yours are very strong." Elena proclaimed, "You see? We are giving hunger! *Hiii*, this hunger." A sister of one of the women I had visited lamented that she had thought her sister was improving: "She was all swollen before, and after taking the pills her body was reducing, she started to return to normal, and we said that she is already better. But it was only to say farewell." This woman had passed away two days earlier because, her sister maintained, there was not enough food. She had died of hunger. The sisters were each eligible for a supplemental food basket from the hospital, but they had not received it in two months. The fact that this woman told me her sister had died of hunger related to ARVs, however, pointed to an established connection between ARVs and hunger that was clear in the minds of at least some community members, and to a tragic paradox in the treatment of AIDS in central Mozambique.

These repeated accounts, particularly the persistent complaint that the medication itself was causing hunger, gave me pause: the description of a "different" hunger that Batista characterized as another illness in itself, Elena's account of treatment "giving" people hunger, the anguish and fear in Madalena's hunger that bites and can kill, the story of the sister who died of hunger while on ARVs, and the suggestions that fear of this hunger kept people from seeking testing and treatment—all these stories spoke to the multiple connections between hunger, HIV/AIDS, and antiretroviral treatment.

HUNGER IN THE AIDS ECONOMY

AIDS and hunger have been linked on multiple levels. When AIDS first emerged in east Africa, it was termed "slim disease" because of the way victims' bodies wasted away.[5] Malnutrition and parasitic coinfection increase susceptibility to infection.[6] In a landmark article, scholars Alex De Waal and Alan Whiteside call the vicious cycle of famine and AIDS in southern Africa the "new variant famine," postulating four factors contributing to worsening food shortages in southern Africa and limiting recovery from HIV/AIDS: physiological interactions between HIV and malnutrition that make the body more susceptible to infection and transmission, household level labor shortages due to adult morbidity and mortality and a related increase in the numbers of dependents, loss of assets and skills due to adult mortality, and an increasing burden of care for sick adults and children orphaned by AIDS.[7]

Hunger in contemporary Mozambique is not necessarily due to the lack of food availability, but rather to the lack of access, as food is increasingly available only through market mechanisms, leaving the poor vulnerable to fluctuations in prices.[8] Chronic malnutrition levels increased from 31 percent in 1997 to 46 percent in 2006.[9] When I began this research, 54 percent of the population lived in extreme poverty, spending less than one dollar per day, and 75 percent of poor family's budgets in urban Manica were spent on food.[10] The dynamics of the new variant famine seemed evident. I accompanied a home-based care volunteer, Augustina, on a visit to a family living in a rural district just outside Chimoio. Unlike in the crowded *bairros* of Chimoio's cane city, homesteads here were disparately spaced, and huts were next to *machambas*. One woman we met, Zinha, had gone to the hospital, where she was given pills. Her ribs were visible in her chest as she raised a thin arm to shake a plastic baggie full of pills: "I take these but they make me feel hungry. I want to eat, but I don't have any food." "But you are surrounded by *machambas*," replied Augustina, pointing to the open land all around. Zinha did have some cucumbers and manioc growing, but she explained she lacked the stamina to work for very long and could not afford to hire anyone. Her husband had died. Inside her hut she had a mosquito net, a small pile of clothes, three ears of corn, two mangos, and a cucumber, as well as some pots and pans that Augustina had brought her and a clay pot (*pendekari*) for preparing corn porridge (*sadza*). Before we departed, Augustina picked some cucumbers and gave her some money for them. As we left Augustina shook her head. "She is afraid of taking those pills without having anything in her stomach. Just cucumber, water? That won't do."

Hunger was integral to the experience of living with HIV/AIDS, and food and livelihood were key to recovery. That is why hunger came up so often in the conversations in the Day Hospital, in associations, and in CHBC networks. A biomedical literature in the area of nutrition, food insecurity, and HIV/AIDS that has emerged since this fieldwork began confirms that these factors are crucial to effectively addressing HIV/AIDS in Africa. This literature elucidates the bidirectional links between food insecurity and HIV/AIDS, as not only can HIV/AIDS lead to food insecurity through lost job income and lost labor for food production on *machambas*, but food insecurity can also lead to HIV acquisition, as those who are malnourished are more vulnerable to disease progression through nutritional, mental health, and behavioral pathways.[11] Clinicians and administrators, however, seemed reluctant to see hunger as inextricably connected to AIDS. Clinicians in the Day Hospital rebuked patients for bringing up hunger as a part of their illness, as well as for bringing their malnourished bodies in for care. They often told their patients they needed to find a way to eat and could not expect the hospital to address all of their problems. Policy makers were concerned that providing food was paternalistic and not sustainable.[12] The latter concern referred to difficulties and expenses associated with the transportation and storage of food aid from the WFP.

The national Working Group on Nutrition and Antiretroviral Treatment, which included representatives of government ministries, donors, and NGOs, met in Maputo during my fieldwork. They hoped they could shift the provision of food onto other government agencies or community organizations. They also discussed providing cash or vouchers for purchasing food in local shops and markets. However, they maintained that "with respect to HIV/AIDS, food should be seen as something that will assist adherence to medications and improving health, not to resolve social problems."[13] The attempt to separate medical from social problems represents a blind spot in the vision of health in these spaces of leadership, particularly in the context of the AIDS epidemic, which is fueled by social and structural factors. Not only were the limited food aid programs not resolving social problems; in some ways they seemed to exacerbate them, by perpetuating an economy of scarcity that provoked intense competition.

THE SPECTACLE OF FOOD AID DISTRIBUTION: EMBODIED HEALTH AND VULNERABILITY

Hunger and food were vexed issues for program administrators and clinic providers. WFP supplements from the clinic were distributed monthly, and during my fieldwork I frequently accompanied Joaquim and Rita to the food distribution warehouse (see Figure 17). Sacks of grain were piled high, each emblazoned with the flag of the donating country and a logo: corn-soy blend from USAID, maize and dry pea beans from Canada, and rice from Algeria. This presentation of the food in nationalized sacks seemed to confirm the impression many had of their country's relative place in the world. Recipients lined up outside, often for several hours, and were called in, four at a time, to help themselves to their allotments, which they scooped up from piles on the floor using empty tin cans. When the

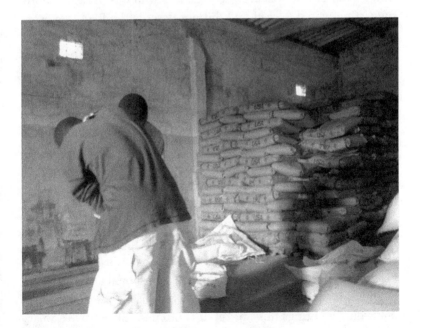

Figure 17. Food distribution warehouse.

piles diminished, a patient would drag a full sack from the back, rip it open, and scoop out the amount. The amounts varied month to month. For example, once there was a surplus of corn-soy blend, so each patient received an entire sack. Another time there was no oil, and many passed up the dry pea beans from Canada because cooking them consumed too much fuel.

The entire process was a very public spectacle, from the queue outside the warehouse to the walk home past neighbors, laden with imported grains. Young men with wheelbarrows gathered outside the warehouse and carried people's allotments to their homes for a few *meticais*. Now and then someone without the WFP ration card that entitled them to a food allotment would squeeze into the warehouse and beseech the coordinator for some grain. Most people who did not have cards were sternly turned away, however. Everyone commented on the bodies of those picking up food—who was fat, who was thin, who was dressed well, and who was in rags—subtly suggesting who deserved and did not deserve the food they were receiving. The potbelly and plump cheeks of one man receiving food stood out from the rest. After seeing how the food was distributed, I sought out Elena to confirm that it was meant to be distributed according to need, for the unemployed and according to anthropometric criteria including body mass index and upper arm circumference.[14] Elena explained that the man was an NHS employee who was also a patient in the Day Hospital and a relative of the coordinator who distributed the WFP cards. She explained that their protocol was to identify the neediest patients as candidates for food supplementation and that this fully employed and clearly well-nourished patient should not be receiving food. While she readily acknowledged the patron-client relationship between the rotund employee and the WFP coordinator, she did not feel this was a legitimate or just use of the scarce food supplements: "We should avoid this kind of abuse. It's not right. We have discussed this before, and it is not only you who brings this up. Yet, it continues." Elena gave a weary shrug. People living with HIV/AIDS saw these contradictions, and even while it did not necessarily surprise anyone, it was nevertheless infuriating. People who looked well nourished used their connections to acquire food, making a mockery of the efforts of the Day Hospital committee on food distribution. Though each household was supposed to receive only one supplemental food basket from any of the multiple sources, many of us knew of many households that received more. Examining people's WFP cards also revealed many received food for more than three months. An association member once remarked to me as the meeting ended: "To get a [WFP] card, one must do a MacGyver" (*tem que fazer um Magaiva*), acquire it through some combination of inventiveness, resourcefulness, and initiative.[15]

Frustrations with food aid often slipped into a discourse of blame and "unworthiness," illustrating a moral economy of development aid. One aid worker complained that she felt the development programs were contributing to a "learned dependence," and that people simply would not work in their *machambas* if they knew they could get food handouts: "These seropositives, they are the hardest people to work with! Always asking for things." A Mozambican accountant, recently hired to work with the association on microcredit projects, explained the challenge he faced:

> Food, that is what they want. If we just distributed food, we would not have space for all the people who would show up. But when I say let's analyze our problems, no one appears. Since independence, the problem with Mozambique, is that we are used to receiving, eating, and insulting the people who give. We have to change this situation.

The coordinator of an AIDS treatment food distribution program remarked: "Those people who don't receive [food] create confusion (*confusão*)!" The term *confusão* is used in political discourse to identify a form of disorder that stands for incivility, chaos, lack of education, crime, and violence.[16] Administrators, providers, and project managers were constantly suspicious, looking for those who tried to illegitimately claim benefits and cause trouble. Some NGOs in Chimoio abandoned their food distribution programs both due to logistical problems and because of concerns that they fostered corruption and deceit. One administrator explained that she felt her organization was constantly trying to establish who, among the groups they served, were the "most vulnerable," while those they visited tried to hide their assets, and often their spouses, in order to appear as poor as possible: "I feel we are supporting the lazy and dishonest." Another NGO stopped its program when it was discovered that some of the food aid was being exported for sale in Zimbabwe. Another suspended its program due to the cost of transporting, storing, and distributing the food. Coordinators from two different organizations explained that while WFP provided US$50 to each organization to cover the cost of distributing each monthly food allotment, they calculated it cost them US$232, and they made up for the difference by paying their employees in rice. When WFP officials discovered this, they suspended the contract. Many of the smaller NGOs preferred not distributing food aid to avoid these complications, but associations of people living with HIV/AIDS prioritized obtaining these contracts. In terms echoing colonial stereotypes, association members were seen as needy but scheming and incapable of being trusted or of thinking beyond the satisfaction of their basic needs. When I asked whether associations could play a greater role in community mobilization and outreach, a hospital provider disagreed: "These associations are too big to help anyone. They are just the same old people, getting fat." These assessments were tinged with judgments of unworthiness.

Association members and people living with HIV were accused of having become accustomed to and dependent on aid programs. Their stated needs were therefore not real and could be dismissed as the result of laziness. In the Day Hospital and NGO food distribution programs, on the other hand, those with too much agency were not deemed worthy of receiving food aid because they were not helpless enough. The search for the worthy beneficiary, the passive and authentic sufferer, the innocent victim that could be saved by humanitarian aid, was fruitless. These individuals and organizations were themselves locked into this cycle, and their own vigilance was constituted by scarcity. Program administrators and policy makers tried to bracket out the social conditions and explicitly medicalize the food as nutritional supplementation meant to be directed toward narrow clinical goals: improving adherence and clinical outcomes. Hunger was officially tied to objective indicators, which themselves shifted over time. Clinical and administrative staff did their best to distribute what they had, but found they had to triage and create additional criteria. Their efforts to distinguish the neediest led to moralizing around hunger. Those who were seen to illegitimately or unnecessarily seek food were accused of sowing disorder (*confusão*) and perpetuating a state of dependence. They were even identified as representing the ills of Mozambique—not that they were poor and HIV positive, but that they were poor, dependent, disorderly, and uneducated.

Ironically, as calls for food grew from people with HIV/AIDS, organizations abandoned their food supplementation programs because they felt overwhelmed and feared they were fostering the evils of dependence. These administrators feared fostering paternalism and unsustainable food supplementation programs. They tried to limit the contexts and purposes in which food supplementation was to be used. Anthropologists James Ferguson and China Scherz remind us that these stances reflect the assumptions of Western Enlightenment philosophies, which equate independence with emancipation and denounce dependence as shameful.[17] These assumptions are reflected in statements such as those of President Guebuza, who blamed hunger and poverty in Mozambique on a lack of "a habit and love for work," blaming the poor for their predicament.[18] With this came the notion that poor Mozambicans had to prove themselves worthy of antiretroviral treatment by demonstrating evidence of an autonomous, independent subjectivity. Ferguson argues, however, that rather than striving for independence, poor people in Africa frequently make "declarations of dependence."[19] Those without means seek to establish hierarchical relations of patronage in which there is a moral imperative for redistribution to maintain the health and harmony of the community. This orientation toward social relations and the collective resonates with a long history of healing in south-eastern Africa, where individual and community well-being are seen as inseparable from each other. Ferguson's provocative point questions the merits and even the possibility of autonomy and independence in an interconnected world. In the AIDS economy, calls for independence and autonomy are tantamount to abandonment and serve as cover for a long-standing neglect of the public's welfare.

"WHO IS EATING IN MY PLACE?"

On World AIDS Day 2005, the governor of Manica province spoke in Chimoio. Citing the increase in AIDS prevalence in the province over the past two years, he asked how it could be possible for the problem to be worsening with 140 different organizations working on HIV. Fátima, the nurse I had accompanied in the Day Hospital, was sitting next to me. She whispered, "Ha, they are all eating the money themselves." It was well known that HIV/AIDS prevention and treatment were not just national but international priorities, with considerable resources being invested in the effort. People living with HIV/AIDS often wondered, if they were still hungry, and if AIDS treatment was a priority: "Where were the resources going? Who is eating in my place?" Fátima seemed to be answering this question when she said the organizations "are eating the money themselves."

The following Saturday morning, I joined a dozen association members listening to a radio broadcast by President Guebuza discussing the national "fight against AIDS" during the Presidential Initiative on HIV/AIDS, a conference held in Maputo with representatives of civil society. A debate arose among us regarding the same issue the governor had pointed to: how HIV prevalence could be worsening despite the efforts of so many organizations and the mobilization of so many resources. Some of those listening to the radio insisted that HIV continued to spread because of poverty, which forced women into unequal sexual relationships and made planning for the future a low priority, with daily survival at stake. Others argued it was ignorance and lack of personal responsibility. The spunky Carmen, whom I knew through the associations, responded to such a comment:

> Look, I *know*. I am taking medications, but I don't have food at home. I've got to go out, talk to people, go looking high and low for a way to feed my children. If someone shows up tomorrow, says, girl, I need to marry you, you will always be happy. What do I do, knowing what I know, living in these conditions, won't I accept? Now tell me is this ignorance or is this poverty?

Carmen bluntly argued that scarcity and need trumped knowledge of risk. Others, however, wondered if the fight against AIDS was being waged in good faith. Gonçalo, the association leader who had easily rattled off the *Vida Positiva* precepts in previous discussions, asked: "If there are so many organizations working on this, why is HIV spreading?" Joel, a young association member whose usual broad smile was replaced by a furrowed brow, called out:

> Go ask the Parliament [of Mozambique]. Ask why they accept that we are dying here in Mozambique? Why won't *you* get fat? It is because so many people are living off of this! Far from trying to get bread because of this disease [as we are], some are living off of it, living off of us!"

Gonçalo related the situation to the experience of the civil war that had ended over a decade before: "Where there is crisis, people get rich. Some die, but others profit; that is quite normal." These comments pointed to the frustrating paradox of how as HIV/AIDS gained prominence and importance as a national issue, the benefits somehow eluded those who suffered from the disease. Even when lifesaving treatment was available, it inflicted hunger even while bringing health.

The question "who is eating in my place?" was directed against a dysfunctional system that offered pills that simultaneously extend life and exacerbate hunger. This language drew on long-standing metaphors of hunger and eating as a language for discussing inequality and illegitimate accumulation and corruption. During the socialist era, a protruding gut characterized the selfish counterrevolutionary cartoon character Xiconhoca, the antithesis of the "new man" of the socialist revolution used in official government propaganda to caricature "enemies of the revolution" (see figures 18, 19, and 20).[20] This

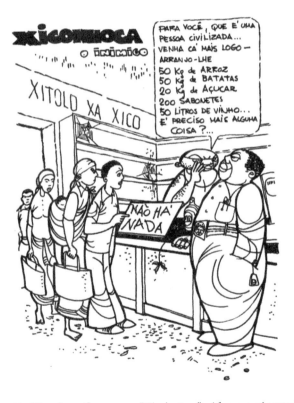

Figure 18. Xiconhoca the enemy; "Xico's store" with a prominent sign for those in line for food reading: "there is nothing" while whispering to his portly friend: "For you, a civilized person, come here later and I'll get you 50 kg of rice, 50 kg of potatoes, 20 kg of sugar, 200 soaps, 50 liters of wine . . . and do you need anything else?" *Source:* FRELIMO (1979).

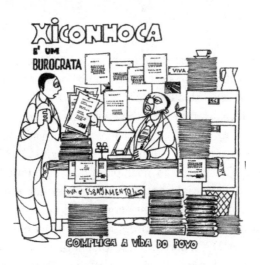

Figure 19. Xiconhoca is a bureaucrat: he complicates the life of the people. *Source:* FRELIMO (1979).

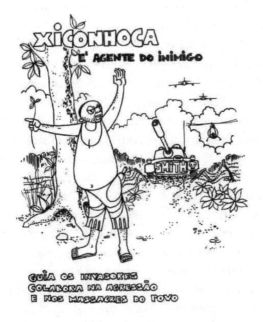

Figure 20. Xiconhoca is an agent of the enemy: he guides the invaders. He collaborates in aggression and the massacre of the people. *Source:* FRELIMO (1979).

symbol of immoral accumulation persists; a headline for a newspaper article critical of government actions against hunger read: "One Does Not Fight Hunger with a Full Belly."[21]

There were fears that only the cleverest, the most resourceful, and the well connected could survive the sinister and shadowy forces that seemed to lie behind the "fight against HIV/AIDS." An atmosphere of distrust and near paranoia surrounded treatment and food aid. Potential beneficiaries were either too needy and dependent or not quite helpless enough to deserve assistance. And who was eating the AIDS resources, eating in place of the people living with HIV/AIDS? There was a suspicion that, while people living with AIDS went hungry, there were others who were getting rich, fueling conspiracy theories about the cure for AIDS being held back in order to enrich foreign organizations or to depopulate Africa. In fact, these suspicions were not entirely unfounded. The majority of HIV/AIDS funds in Mozambique did go to private and foreign organizations, and pharmaceutical firms investing in AIDS treatment found their profits growing.[22] PEPFAR provided $200–400 million annually, the equivalent of the total budget of the entire Ministry of Health, but nearly all of this sum flowed "off budget" to US NGOs and contractors, partly due to structural adjustment–mandated public spending constraints.[23] Thus, while Mozambique received substantial funding for AIDS, much of this was "phantom aid" that flowed right back to American organizations rather than being invested in the Mozambican health infrastructure.[24] Donors and philanthropists could congratulate themselves and each other on their compassion and generosity and on the individual lives they saved, but my informants pointed to their hunger and their economic problems when I asked them about the pills they were taking and the epidemic they faced.

In this respect, we might wonder along with frontline AIDS workers if the "business of AIDS" did not function as a virulent form of neocolonial extraction, providing foreign organizations with jobs; expanding programs that relied on the expertise and the largesse of foreign organizations; enlisting cohorts of African patients in regimes of lifetime treatment; and benefiting from the voluntary, poorly compensated labor of the underemployed. Antiretrovirals and WFP baskets functioned as postcolonial palliatives, while the rich continued to eat the poor. These observations are consonant with historian of Africa Nancy Rose Hunt's description of "extraction" and "salvation" as the main historical modes of northern intervention in Africa.[25] These dynamics were readily apparent during the colonial area, and they persist in contemporary global health interventions such as the AIDS treatment scale-up.

This situation results from the reinforcing blind spots of contemporary neoliberal development and individually oriented biomedicine.[26] By targeting a biological condition and placing the responsibility for health and well-being in the hands of the individual, political and economic concerns were sidelined and the roots of the AIDS epidemic in inequality and structural violence were rendered invisible. Histories of colonialism and the racialized oppression that established the conditions for the AIDS pandemic were disregarded as the onus for treatment was put on individuals and families. Alternative forms of solidarity were undermined as disease-related distinctions determined eligibility for scarce resources. This supports the criticism that the focus on keeping bodies alive with pharmaceuticals leaves people vulnerable when humanitarian interventions and saving lives displace a politics that can address economic inequalities and social justice.[27]

LEARNING FROM PEOPLE LIVING WITH HIV/AIDS

Lifesaving medicines in the context of postcolonial neoliberal inequality exposed people to the brutality of their poverty in new and painful ways, through the irony of eating only ARVs when food itself could indeed have been considered medicine. By working toward narrow aims, quantified at the level of individual lives saved and numbers of patients attended to, the treatment interventions effectively disarticulated HIV/AIDS from social and economic realities. Illness was reframed in terms of personal responsibility and tied to individual behaviors and risk factors, creating a tendency to blame that some argue represents an additional health burden, the "double burden" of neoliberalism.[28] Rather than conceiving of health and recovery as individual notions, this book points to the importance of supportive social networks as constitutive of health and recovery. In her work on AIDS in Uganda, Susan Reynolds Whyte points out, "Food and eating together are both an entitlement and an expression of personal concern and attention, and sharing is both a value and a tactic. Sharing food is about caring, as both practice and metaphor."[29] On the other hand, eating alone and not sharing food with others communicates antisocial sentiment and is understood to be a defining trait of witches, distinguished by unbridled self-interest and greed.[30] This metaphor provides a framework for understanding hunger as embodying the inequalities and injustices people in the treatment programs perceived and experienced, even as their lives were being saved. Rita and Joaquim managed to benefit from ARVs and associations, but they were able to build their own support structure through their church, where Rita became a healer herself. Long waits and treatment delays led many others, like Teresa, to choose the *n'anga* as part of the eclectic therapeutic milieu that sought to repair the social relationships integral to material support. While this ended tragically for Teresa, her ability to choose was severely constrained by structural factors such as her financial dependence on her husband. But she did exercise agency in choosing dignity over degradation and the available care of the *n'anga* over the chaos and illogic of the Day Hospital. The *n'anga* also offered a form of care that was simply not available in the Day Hospital, oriented toward harmonizing the social relationships Teresa relied on. We would do well to recognize the logic of Teresa's actions rather than dismiss them as products of ignorance. This is not to idealize the *n'anga* or dismiss the potential of ARVs to have extended

Teresa's life. My point is that ARVs are a much more effective treatment in the context of robust social support.

Associations provided a staunch support system, a safe place for exchange and recovery where members stitched together biomedical knowledge, *Vida Positiva*, and Pentecostal healing practices. Association activists like Elena, Florência, and Gonçalo took the tenets of positive living seriously, and they benefited from the robust support available to them in the early days of the scale-up. The individual-focused aspects of *Vida Positiva*, with its emphasis on proper lifestyle, such as abstinence or monogamy with a condom, adequate sleep, balanced diet, sobriety, planning for the future, and shunning the *n'anga*, had an elective affinity with emergent forms of Pentecostalism, which similarly advocated a break with the past, individual morality, and salvation through grace. Both Pentecostalism and *Vida Positiva* valorized a cosmopolitan, educated, modern outlook and resonated with neoliberal notions of individual autonomy and entrepreneurialism. The figure of the modern, independent, and educated AIDS patient emerged as the ideal of *Vida Positiva* and was the standard that people living with AIDS were asked to live up to in the AIDS economy. While Elena, Florência, and Gonçalo could be counted among those who were "saved" through *Vida Positiva* and ARVs, it was not just medication and behavioral change that helped them, but food aid, steady employment, and vibrant social support systems of kin and peers who were living with AIDS. While some of the associations I encountered in Mozambique were engaged in programs that bolstered livelihood, including providing food, when these associations could not sustain their growing membership many, such as Takashinga, became sites of competition and accusation. An ideology that prioritized individual over collective interests and responsibilities—and the need to prove oneself worthy of treatment amid scarcity of food and livelihood opportunities—led to division and alienation.

In the wake of the austerity measures of structural adjustment, voluntary labor stood in for a functioning health system. CHBC volunteers like Arminda brought their skills and dedication to caring for those suffering from HIV/AIDS who lacked adequate treatment, and their patients expressed their gratitude. Yet the organizations benefiting from their labor, such as Mufudzi, exploited the volunteers' unpaid labor while extolling their altruism and "community empowerment." CHBC volunteers sought to be a part of a mutually collaborative community of care providers, but as the scale-up proceeded and increasingly focused on administering medication to individuals, they were marginalized. The community-based vanguards of the AIDS treatment, the associations and the CHBC networks, that were used to launch the initial phase of the treatment scale-up, were largely cast aside, as were the hopes and aspirations of the activists and volunteers who laid the groundwork for the scale-up. Arminda's own unrealized vision of solidarity and mutual support spoke to alternative relationships and power structures, of mutual accountability, recognition, and interdependence. While she provided compassionate care and accompaniment, the arrival of ARVs seemed to render her no longer necessary, despite her years of devotion and dedication.

The Day Hospital made some promising attempts to support individuals and families, through the *testemunha* protocol and the *agentes terapêuticos*, which provided not only counseling but also employment to people living with AIDS. Critics of the Day Hospital system argued that AIDS-specific specialty services created internal inequities in the health system, consuming resources that could benefit the entire health system. Physician-anthropologist Arthur Kleinman has observed that practitioners of biomedicine "experience a therapeutic environment in which the traditional moral goals of healing have been replaced by narrow technical and bureaucratic objectives."[31] In Mozambique's AIDS treatment scale-up, the result was that high adherence rates were prioritized over the very lives of patients. Even those who managed to receive treatment, such as Florência, were plagued by a harrowing hunger caused by their medications. Health-care providers and administrators either blamed the patient for hunger, discounted it, or medicalized it. When, in the name of efficiency and equity, the Day Hospitals were shut down in favor of integration of AIDS care into the general NHS, the position of *agente terapêutico* was discontinued, as were the *testemunha* protocol and the support of associations. In this way, the fears that patients would be abandoned by the health system were realized.

While there is clearly no magic bullet solution for AIDS in Mozambique, there is much to learn from the experiences of people living with AIDS in the early days of the treatment scale-up. Despite the promise of the initial scale-up, the fact that the treatment inflicted rather than resolved hunger led to a sense of disappointment, if not betrayal. The AIDS scale-up, with its orientation toward the individual and a specific kind of forward-looking, self-interested subject to the exclusion of all others, was actually pathogenic.

FROM GLOBAL HEALTH TO GLOBAL SOCIAL MEDICINE

Structural adjustment programs of the early 1980s attacked the state as totalitarian, inefficient, and corrupt and promised liberation through the market. Despite the negative consequences worldwide, private, technical, disease-focused intervention remains the dominant model for global health. With the withdrawal of states from the business of providing housing, education, and medical services, well-meaning NGOs offering practical stopgaps are instrumentalized by neoliberal policies that declare everything and every service to be for sale. As physician-anthropologist Sam Dubal writes, even a model NGO such as Partners in Health (PIH), which advocated for the global AIDS treatment scale-up, was attacked by rebels in Peru, who saw the NGO's collaboration with the authoritarian government as a component of that government's counterinsurgency campaign, which opposed radical equality of the poorest groups in Peru.[32]

Much of today's global health is underwritten by the wealthiest individuals and corporations in the world. The Bill and Melinda Gates Foundation has come to set the global agenda in health, nutrition, agriculture, development, and education, favoring a "neutral" technical and private approach to producing and shaping knowledge, organizations, and strategies in these areas.[33] Such institutions espouse what anthropologist Tobias Rees describes as a stateless vision of a humanity bound by a common biology.[34] While the nation-state does not have a long history of benevolence in Mozambique, my own glimpses of this vision of a stateless biological humanity reveal it to be decidedly dystopian, resulting in marginalization, exclusion, and alienation, a paradoxical world in which sometimes the only way to survive is by having a chronic illness.[35] The philanthro-capitalism fueling many technologically intensive, privatized global health initiatives depends on profits amassed through exploitation, speculation, and expropriation.[36] Unlike public institutions, private organizations are accountable to nobody but their boards and share-holders, threatening democratic global health governance and scientific independence.[37]

This book began by noting the AIDS treatment scale-up has been celebrated as the signature triumph of the "new global health." This claim was put forth by distinguished medical historian Allan Brandt, who argued in *The New England Journal of Medicine* that the AIDS response had disrupted old thinking in international health, challenging the divisions between prevention and treatment, between public health and biomedical intervention. It initiated a new era of health activism and triggered unprecedented investments in health that led to the creation of new public, private, and philanthropic global health institutions. The overall approach foregrounded a human rights framework that recognized ethical and moral values such as equity as central to prevention and treatment of disease.[38] While global AIDS activism is a powerful example of the potential of direct action and mass mobilization to shift policy at the highest levels, particularly in the ways activists rebuked the homophobia and racism that often prevented effective action, the case of central Mozambique that this book explores indicates how partial and limited these successes have been for many in the world.[39] The new global health infrastructure—privatized and dependent on the largesse of billionaire philanthrocapitalists—represents an unwelcome continuity with the past and a move in the wrong direction, as public sector health and social welfare systems continue to be eroded.[40] Despite fifteen years of major increased foreign aid for health from donors, Mozambique has not experienced expanded access to health services, because the majority of this money goes to foreign NGOs and consultants. In many ways, the AIDS treatment effort retrenched the logics and structures of inequality that preceded the AIDS epidemic.

Richard Horton, the editor of the influential medical journal *The Lancet*, characterized Brandt's thesis as a "dangerous myth," arguing that global health did not start with the response to the HIV/AIDS pandemic, but rather events preceding it by at least thirty years: "Global health is about power and poverty, violence and exploitation, oppression and silence, and collusion and exclusion. If one views global health using this broader lens, the historical turn that was the decisive and creative moment for the birth of global health was surely decolonization. It was decolonization, beginning in the 1950s with legacies that continue to this day, which illuminated the myriad pressures that shape the health of peoples worldwide."[41] It is not new technologies, novel funding structures, disciplinary shifts, or billionaire philanthrocapitalists that should drive global health, but broad movements that seek justice and equity for all.

The concepts of structural competency and structural vulnerability have been proposed by scholars and physicians who seek to revitalize a social medicine that explicitly attends to social, economic, and political determinants of health in the clinic and in global health.[42] They draw on the historical examples of physician-anthropologist-politician Rudolph Virchow, who in 1848 responded to a typhus epidemic in Upper Silesia by calling for full employment, higher wages, the establishment of agricultural cooperatives, and universal education, and Frantz Fanon, the psychiatrist and revolutionary whose calls for decolonization can be read as the first manifestos for global health.[43] These approaches foreground social histories, housing, employment, discrimination based on race and gender, colonialism, imperialism, and related factors in order to identify the ways social structures make people sick, positioning disease as the very embodiment of these structures.

Practically, such an approach entails humility and the recognition of the limits of clinical medicine alongside a willingness to collaborate across forms of expertise and class. Such a social medicine would seek to intervene not only "Where There Is No Doctor," as the title of the classic manual directs us, but also as anthropologist Kenneth Maes suggests, "Where There Is No Labor Movement."[44] Anthropologist James Pfeiffer has called for a reinvestment in "the well-known fundamentals" of public institutions, services, and safety nets rather than the technological innovation sought by the captains of philanthrocapitalism.[45] Pfeiffer and his colleagues' work in Mozambique over the past decades show that there are ways to work around the neoliberal consensus, such as developing the NGO Code of Conduct for Health Systems Strengthening and by participating with like-minded partners in a "sector-wide approach" to public systems strengthening that explicitly aims to work around the fiscal austerity policies that strangle the health system.[46] Yet the current NGO-dominated health system impedes progress toward universal health coverage in settings like Mozambique.[47] These approaches call us to go beyond saving lives to rebuilding institutions and workforces and working toward universal health coverage on a global scale.[48]

A truly collaborative and holistic global health should be guided not by an individualistic biomedical and neoliberal approach, but by an ethics of interdependence, which recognizes that inequality and injustice are socially corrosive and detrimental to individual and collective health.[49] Such an ethics would value inclusion, social support, and solidarity above competition and individual autonomy.

This approach would echo the relational view of disease and care prevalent in central Mozambique, one that recognizes that social commitments—rather than isolated individual behaviors or technological innovations—truly determine health and collective survival.

These ideals can readily be concretized in specific policies and practices. The early days of the treatment scale-up discussed in this book reveal that in order for AIDS treatment to truly be successful, it needs to go beyond providing medication to those who can regularly attend the clinic. This would include making the treatment as accessible as possible to as many people as possible by extending the health system to meet the needs of all Mozambican citizens. Individualized medical treatment must be offered within a robust and fully functional universal health-care system. It would also include providing food as a treatment every bit as necessary to survival as ARVs. Well-compensated and well-trained community health work should be a health intervention in and of itself, rather than a cheap means to the shortsighted end of meeting goals of numbers cared for, tested, and treated. It would also mean supporting community-based initiatives such as associations of people living with HIV/AIDS, as well as taking seriously the expressed needs of these groups and individuals with lived experience of HIV/AIDS.

Many practical strategies have been suggested for improving AIDS treatment in Mozambique that are consistent with these recommendations:

provide food supplementation to all patients enrolled in care, as well as farming cooperatives and home garden collectives;[50]

improve provider accountability and performance and empower patients;[51]

collaborate with nonbiomedical healers;[52] and

engage "expert" patients to support and educate new patients.[53]

Good ideas and promising models exist, but the challenge is implementing them in a political climate oriented toward privatization, market-based solutions, scaling up the one-size-fits-all best practice, and an emphasis on new and improved technology.[54] To be broadly effective, interventions must go beyond technical fixes and targeted benefits. Targeted benefits can have a corrosive effect. In a context such as Mozambique, where 70 percent of the population is poor, a targeted entitlement program risks leading to social division, and this is precisely what happened in the AIDS economy. The scarcity of food and livelihood opportunities led to competition and alienation.

In order to assure health for all, not just for those living with HIV/AIDS, a robust, adequately funded and staffed national health system is fundamental. Additionally, a universal program providing livelihood support, such as South Africa's Basic Income Grant, is also needed, as the majority struggle to subsist.[55] There is growing momentum for the establishment of a global social protection fund, which would help finance national social protection floors that would include universal access to essential health care and basic income security.[56] These programs provide a minimum basic income and standard of living to all and have been shown to alleviate poverty and stimulate local economies in Mozambique as well as other settings.[57] They are an effort to build an inclusive economy in which all can rely on being able to satisfy their basic needs for survival. Moving in this direction requires income redistribution and reforming the global taxation regime, which allows multinational corporations and wealthy individuals to hide their income from taxation while undermining the capacity of states to provide social protection.[58] It also requires moving away from a neocolonial extractive model of economic development. Indeed, following through on Horton's call for a global health based in decolonization would entail working toward reparations for colonialism and slavery.[59] Perhaps universal social protections could be funded through a mechanism that taxes those who have profited from colonialism, slavery, and genocide.

AIDS funding plateaued in 2010. While mortality due to AIDS has decreased, HIV prevalence has continued to rise in Mozambique, especially among the poor and women.[60] The simmering discontent about hunger that I encountered in my fieldwork proved to be prescient and widespread, as rising food, fuel, and utility costs sparked revolts in urban centers throughout the country from 2008 to 2012.[61] Violence has resurfaced in recent years over widespread discontent with a government unable to thwart growing poverty and inequality and an extractive model of economic development that benefits very few Mozambicans.[62] The prevalence of HIV alongside extreme poverty speaks to the ongoing disaster of neoliberal policy for health and well-being in Mozambique.

This book goes to press in the shadow of a new global pandemic, COVID-19. The SARS-CoV-2 virus may be unprecedented in the speed and scale of its transmission, but the pandemic is chillingly similar to HIV/AIDS in the ways it has both tracked the fault lines of social inequality to target the marginalized and the dispossessed and revealed the hollowness of the contemporary global health rhetoric of equity.[63] Like HIV/AIDS, COVID-19 is already threatening devastating economic impacts and leading to yet another "new-variant" famine.[64] COVID-19 exacerbates the ongoing stress of the HIV/AIDS pandemic and neoliberal austerity, creating a new hazard that additionally hampers efforts to survive the preexisting conditions.[65] COVID-19 makes the lessons set forth in this book all the more urgent, in that biomedical tunnel vision must be avoided and wider socioeconomic and health inequities must be addressed in a proactive, lasting manner. This is an opportunity to erect some of the structures of solidarity, commitment, and accountability that we need for an effective and ethical global social medicine.

In writing this book, I am trying to make good on my obligation to the many Mozambicans who shared their stories with me in the hopes that they might bring about some change. This book has attempted to chart the lives of individuals and institutions in the thick of the Mozambican AIDS epidemic during a key moment in Mozambique and global health at the turn of the twenty-first century. Hunger, the reality and the metaphor, points to many of the dynamic tensions that permeated life in Mozambique during the AIDS treatment scale-up.

In central Mozambique, programs that focused primarily on the distribution of ARVs exacerbated suffering and increased social conflict and competition. While treatment for AIDS became more available, overall biomedical coverage did not increase, and living conditions worsened as the basic problems of hunger and economic citizenship were not addressed. The interventions could attain their stated and measured goals, while the "beneficiaries" of the programs continued to suffer in an environment of weakening social solidarity. The clarion critique of "all I eat is ARVs!" is a reminder that the technological magic bullet of ARVs alone is an insufficient intervention in the face of the increasing hunger and inequalities that continue unabated in contemporary Mozambique.

Acknowledgments

This book has had a long period of gestation over my training in anthropology, medicine, and psychiatry and my initial years on faculty. It began as my doctoral dissertation in the University of California, Berkeley, and UC San Francisco Joint Program in Medical Anthropology, with Philippe Bourgois, Vincanne Adams, Nancy Scheper-Hughes, and Vinh-Kim Nguyen serving as my committee. They have each continued to support this project as it has developed as well as support me as a scholar. I may never have pursued the PhD without the encouragement of Harvey Weinstein, who mentored me when I was a medical student in the UCB-UCSF Joint Medical Program. Judith Justice has been a steady source of encouragement since my first days as a graduate student.

Many of my classmates in medical anthropology who offered early assistance and collaboration have become friends and colleagues, particularly Seth Holmes, Scott Stonington, Johanna Crane, Thurka Sangaramoorthy, Jennifer Liu, and China Scherz. Thurka and Jennifer formed the core of a virtual dissertation writing group that grew to include Adia Benton and Elise Carpenter.

Funding for this project came from the UCSF School of Medicine Rainer's Fund, the UCB Center for African Studies Andrew and Mary

Thompson Rocca Scholarship, a Foreign Language and Area Studies Award, the Fulbright-Hayes Doctoral Dissertation Research Award, the UC President's Dissertation Year Fellowship, the Roskilde University Guest PhD Fellowship, the UCSF International Program Grant, the UCSF Clinical and Translational Research Fellowship, and the American Council of Learned Societies Fellowship.

Many people and organizations in Mozambique opened their doors and their lives to me over many years, and while I cannot thank them by name due to confidentiality concerns, this project and book would have been impossible without their generosity and sincerity—*maitabassa maningue*! I thank everyone who took the time to speak to me and in many cases develop relationships that have lasted for years. I especially thank all those who appear in this book with pseudonyms. Those whom I call Arminda, Adélia, Diogo, Elena, Fernando, Gonçalo, Isabela, Lucia, Mayita, Oswaldo, Pedro, Rita, and Joaquim have been especially integral to teaching me about Mozambique and the AIDS economy over the years. Those whom I call Bruno, Carmen, Clara, Eusebio, Fátima, Florência, Joel, Julia, Luiz, Severino, Suraia, Suzana, and Teresa all generously made time for me in their work and their lives.

For their advice and guidance throughout the project, but especially at the beginning stages, I'd like to thank Alfredo Vergara, Julie Cliff, Sandy McGunnegill, Jose Caetano, Felisbela Gaspar, Kenny Sherr, Sarah Gimbel, Mary Anne Mercer, Steve Gloyd, James Pfeiffer, Wendy Prosser, Mark Micek, Carina Winberg, Petros Nyakunu, Ernesto Pechisso, Dr. Jaqueta, Diedericke Geelhoed, Wendy Johnson, Pablo Montoya, and Clara Chinacaj. For helping me get settled in Mozambique, I'd like to thank Alexandre Lourenço, Maria Ana Chadreque Correia, Suzanne Smith, Stephan Spatt, Claudia Szivatz, and Alejandro Soto.

Ana Rita Boane provided indispensable support in translation and navigation of central Mozambique. I have benefited from engagements with colleagues who also conduct research in Mozambique, including Julie Cliff, Jason Sumich, Juan Obarrio, Rosa Williams, Christie Schuetze, Erling Høg, Carla Braga, Ramah McKay, Joel Christian Reed, and Bent Steenberg Olsen. I was fortunate to share my fieldsite with Michael Walker, who has been a vital source of expertise and friendship. James Pfeiffer and Rachel Chapman have fundamentally shaped my understanding of Mozambique and of global health, both in terms of what it is and what it could be.

Lisa Richey provided support and feedback during my time as a dissertation writing fellow in Roskilde. I also received valuable feedback from the students and faculty at Roskilde during my time there. I have learned from my collaborations with Kenneth Maes and Svea Closser on the politics of community health worker programs and with Adia Benton and Thurka Sangaramoorthy on the temporality of positive living. The African Studies writing group I was a part of at the University of Washington during my psychiatry residency helped me begin the process of turning the dissertation into a book; thank you to Lynn Thomas, Johanna Crane, Ben Gardner, Ron Krabill, Nora Kenworthy, and Danny Hoffman. Meg Stalcup, Gaymon Bennett, and Roger Brent brought me into a supportive space at the Center for Biological Futures at the Fred Hutchinson Cancer Research Center to do this work while I was in psychiatry residency training. Thank you to Deborah Cowley and Jurgen Unützer for supporting my work on this project while I was a resident, and to Ken Wells for supporting it when I was a Robert Woods Johnson Clinical Scholar and as a member of the UCLA-VA Center for Excellence on Veteran Resilience and Recovery.

I completed the book manuscript in the vibrant intellectual community I've been fortunate to be a part of at UCLA as a faculty member, between the Center for Social Medicine and Humanities, the Department of Anthropology, the International Institute, and the West Los Angeles VAMC. Hannah Appel was instrumental in guiding me to key sources of support. Joel Braslow has been a key advocate and mentor. The student, resident, and faculty participants of the clinical ethnography seminar in the Center for Social Medicine and Humanities provided very helpful feedback on a late draft of the manuscript. During the past few years, Liza Buchbinder, Kim Sue, Jennifer Karlin, Yvonne Yang, Roya Ijadi-Maghsoodi, and Jared Greenberg have provided moral support throughout the often-lonely process of writing.

I have presented parts of this work in the UCLA Medicine, Mind, and Culture seminar and received valuable feedback from students and faculty there. I have also presented in the Arizona State University School of Historical, Philosophical, and Religious Studies; the University of Washington Department of Anthropology; the UC Berkeley Center for Social Medicine; and the UCSF Department of Anthropology, History, and Social Medicine, and at the Symposium on AIDS, Citizenship and Governance in Southern Africa, the Social Impacts of the ARV Scale-up Meeting at Columbia University, and the Religious Engagements with AIDS in Africa conference, as well as on panels at the meetings of the American Anthropological Association; the Society for Medical Anthropology; the African Studies Association; the Society for the Social Studies of Science; and the Society

for Humanities, Social Science, and Medicine. I appreciate the feedback
and discussion with the organizers and participants at all of these events
and am grateful to have been a part of them.

The manuscript benefited from close readings and detailed feedback
from Claire Wendland, Adia Benton, and two additional anonymous
reviewers, as well as the faculty board of UC Press. Laurie Hart's tremen-
dous breadth of knowledge and nuanced reflections facilitated improvements. Sam Dubal was extraordinarily generous in reading multiple
drafts and in offering perceptive, detailed criticism. Francisco Saidane
and Michael Walker provided help with Chitewe terms. The editorial
assistance of Lisa Moore, at Glen Hollow, *Ink.*, brought coherence to what
often felt like a tangled mess of words and emotion. I am not sure I ever
would have finished without her contributions. I am grateful to Naomi
Schneider for including this book in the University of California Press
public anthropology series and for patiently shepherding it to completion.
I was fortunate to benefit from the mentorship of Philippe Bourgois at the
project's inception, when he was my dissertation chair, and then again at its
conclusion, as a colleague and friend. His critically engaged anthropology
is a sterling example of scholarship in the service of pragmatic change.

Throughout my travels and extended training, my family has been a
steady source of faith, optimism, and care. Thanks to my parents, Dionysios and Vanna-Maria; my brothers, Potouli and Alexandros; my sisters-
in-law, Karen and Hilliary; my parents-in-law, Jackie and David; and my
brother-in-law, Bill. My partner and wife, Katy Krantz, deserves thanks
for accompanying this work from near and from afar, for inspiring me to
create, and for always believing in me. Our children, Dionysios and Yianna,
are younger than this project, and their creative energy and keen observations have been a continual source of sustenance and joy.

The greatest thanks go to those in Mozambique who invited me into
their lives and shared their experiences and visions of illness, health, and
healing.

Glossary

Most terms listed here are of Portuguese origin. Origins other than Portuguese are specified in applicable entries.

Agentes Polivalentes Elementares (APEs)   Community health workers trained in the 1970s in independent Mozambique's first national health-care system. They were recruited from within the community and received six months of training to provide basic preventative education, basic medications, and first aid care.

agentes terapêuticos   Official title of the peer adherence counselors who were people living with HIV/AIDS and worked in the Day Hospital.

aldeamento   Communal villages constructed by the Portuguese colonial state for strategic reasons during the war for independence.

assimilado   Mozambican native who was granted the status of Portuguese citizen through religious conversion and educational attainment. See also Indigenato.

azar   Misfortune, bad luck, or cursed fate, which could be sent via witchcraft or an evil spirit.

bairro   Neighborhood, quarter, or section of town.

biscate   Odd job, short-term work.

botânica   Literally medicine; refers to a substance used to cure and
   protect in the context of healing, but to poison and destroy in the
   context of sorcery. See also *mutombo* and *droga.*
Cabeça do Velho   "Old Man's Head," nickname for Mount Bengo, a
   landmark commonly associated with the city of Chimoio.
capulana   Colorful cloth worn by women as a wrap and used to carry
   babies and transport goods.
chapa   Minibus, most common mode of transportation on Mozambique's
   streets and highways.
cidade de caniço   "Cane city," neighborhoods surrounding the cement city
   where the majority of residents live, named for the characteristic
   thatched roofs of most of the dwellings.
cidade de cimento   "Cement city," the former colonial city, now often the
   center of contemporary Mozambican cities.
civilizado   The settler citizen of the Portuguese colony, entitled to full
   citizenship rights and living under metropolitan civil law. See also
   Indigenato.
confusão   Term used in political discourse to identify a form of disorder
   that stands for incivility, chaos, lack of education, crime, and violence.
crente   Believer, member of a church.
deslocados   "The displaced"; refers to people who were displaced, chiefly
   from Central Mozambique to the neighboring countries Zimbabwe and
   Malawi, by the civil war between Frelimo and Renamo, between 1978
   and 1992.
doença prolongada   Prolonged illness, often used as a euphemism for AIDS.
doença do século   Disease of the century, used to refer to AIDS.
doente   Patient or sick person.
dom   Spiritual gift of healing.
droga   Literally medicine; refers to a substance used to cure and protect
   in the context of healing, but to poison and destroy in the context of
   sorcery. See also *mutombo* and *bôtanica.*
Esperança   Hope; pseudonym for an association of people living with
   HIV/AIDS.
espírito mau   Evil spirit.
estamos juntos   "We are together," a popular slogan of solidarity from the
   independence movement that has endured to the present day.
esteira   A straw mat used to sit or sleep on.
Estrada Nacional 6   National Highway 6, the highway entering Chimoio.
igreja   Church.

indígena   Indigenous, the category the Portuguese created for native subjects who lived under African law and the particular laws of the individual colonies. See also Indigenato.

Indigenato   The bifurcated Portuguese colonial legal system that defined the difference between settler citizen, or *civilizado*, and native subject, *indígena*.

machamba   Plots of land used for agricultural purposes. Urban families rely on them to supplement their diets and income.

mãe   "Mother," part of the title of Mufudzi CHBC volunteers.

massemba   A relish made with leafy greens (Chitewe).

matembe   Dried fish (Chitewe).

Ministério da Saúde (MISAU)   Ministry of Health.

Missão de Fé Apostólica   Apostolic Faith Mission, one of the oldest Pentecostal churches in southern Africa, with roots in the Azusa Street Revival of Los Angeles, CA.

mupfukwa   Avenging spirit, especially the spirit of the victim of murder or war, who might return to settle a score (Chitewe).

mutombo   Literally medicine; refers to a substance used to cure and protect in the context of healing, but to poison and destroy in the context of sorcery (Chitewe). This is also referred to in Portuguese as *botânica* or *droga*.

muzungu   White foreigner (Chitewe).

n'anga   Traditional healer-diviner (Chitewe); also *curandeiro/a* in Portuguese.

nipa   Homemade liquor, often distilled from fermented corn with sugar.

Operação Produção   Operation Production, a policy applied in 1983 that forcibly removed urban residents deemed unproductive, which included so-called prostitutes, vagrants, and traditional and religious authorities, to forced labor and reeducation camps in the rural north.

palestra   Educational presentation.

pendekari   Clay pot for preparing *sadza* over a cooking fire (Chitewe).

Pense na Vida! Evite SIDA!   "Think of Life! Avoid AIDS!" Slogan used in early AIDS education campaigns.

picada   Footpath.

piringaniso   A spiritual affliction caused after a death in the family when a couple engages in sexual relations before the completion of funeral services. Either the couple or another vulnerable family member could be stricken by the illness. The illness presents with similar constitutional symptoms as AIDS: loss of strength (*kupera simba*), loss of appetite (*kusada kudya*), nausea (*kushotwa*), and fever (*kupisa mwiri*, literally hot body). (Chitewe)

Praça dos Trabalhadores   Worker's Plaza in Chimoio, marked by a vertical concrete slab depicting two stick figures clasping each other's shoulders, each raising a hoe toward a red star above them; a monument from Mozambique's socialist period. Emblematic of the changing times, an addition was made recently in red paint on the base of the monument: "Mozambican Workers Engaged in the Fight Against HIV/AIDS" (*Trabalhadores Moçambicanos Na Luta Contra O HIV/SIDA*).

profete   Healer or diviner of an African Independent Church.

quintal   Front yard.

sadza   Porridge made of corn, sorghum, cassava, or rice; the staple food for lunch and dinner throughout southeastern Africa (Chitewe).

secretário do bairro   "Secretary of the neighborhood," a neighborhood level political leader in the formal postindependence governance structure.

SIDA Mata   "AIDS Kills," slogan used in early AIDS education campaigns.

Sociedade Algodeira de Portugal (SOALPO)   The Cotton Society of Portugal, founded in Portugal in 1944. Chimoio was chosen as one of the society's factory sites because of its location in the Beira corridor; the proximity of the railway and rivers for hydroelectric power; and the burgeoning European settlement, with at the time around a thousand Europeans living in Chimoio.

Sociedade Hidro-Eléctrica do Revuè (SHER)   Hydroelectric Society of the Revuè, established at the same time as SOALPO, which consisted of a hydroelectric dam that supplied first the factory and then later the entire region with electrical power.

Takashinga   "We Were Brave," pseudonym for an association of people living with HIV/AIDS (Chitewe).

técnico de medicina   Nonphysician clinicians working for the National Health Service. They have two and a half to three years of clinical training, compared to six for physicians.

testemunha   Witness, someone a patient has designated to support them in their ARV treatment.

tratamento observado direitamente (TOD)   Directly observed treatment, a protocol whereby the patient must be observed ingesting medication, either in the clinic or at home.

uroi   Sorcery or witchcraft. See also *fetiço* (Chitewe).

vadzimu   ancestral spirits, plural (Chitewe).

Vida Positiva   Living positively.

Xiconhoca   A slovenly, pot-bellied cartoon character popular during the revolution, the embodiment of the antitheses of the "revolutionary man"; his selfishness and doubtful moral conduct risked undermining the entire project of social transformation (Chishangana).

zwirwere zwemunjanji   Sexually transmitted disease, literally "disease from the railway," so named because migrant workers brought these diseases home when they returned from the Rhodesian mines (Chitewe).

zvirwere zvepabonde   Sexually transmitted disease, literally "disease from the sleeping mat" (Chitewe).

Notes

1. MISAU (2005).

2. In his 2013 article, "How AIDS Invented Global Health," preeminent historian of medicine Allan Brandt (2013) characterizes the new global health that emerged as a result of global AIDS efforts as recognizing the supranational character of disease and responses to disease, being based on a knowledge of the burden of disease to identify key disparities, recognizing that people affected by a disease have a role in the discovery and advocacy of new modes of treatment and prevention, and being based on ethical and moral values recognizing that equity and rights are central to the larger goals of preventing and treating illness.

3. UNAIDS (2013).

4. TARV is the Portuguese acronym that health-care providers and patients used to refer to antiretroviral treatment and to the antiretroviral medications themselves. The acronym was pronounced as a word, "tarv," which I translate to the equivalent English initialism ARVs. *Lazarus effect* was introduced in a 1996 *Newsweek* article on the advent of antiretroviral therapy and was used by early advocates of global treatment scale-up (Farmer 1999, 264; Koenig, Leandre, and Farmer 2004). Whyte (2014)

wrote that stories of the Lazarus effect were told in Uganda to "amaze, reassure, and convince" when treatment was still new. Prince (2016) provides a social history of the imagery of the Lazarus effect and discusses the ways it operated in western Kenya.

5. Richey and Ponte (2011) critically examined the use of the Lazarus effect imagery for marketing Product Red, an effort to link consumer spending to AIDS treatment in southern Africa.

6. See a critical discussion of the notion of "the end of AIDS" in Kenworthy, Thomann, and Parker (2017).

7. Feierman (1985).

8. Collins (2006).

9. Matsinhe (2005, 35).

10. Collins (2006).

11. MISAU (2005).

12. Gray (2013); Messac and Prabhu (2013); D'Adesky (2006).

13. Oomman, Bernstein, and Rosenzweig (2007, 25).

14. Pfeiffer and Chapman (2019).

15. Oomman, Bernstein, and Rosenzweig (2007).

16. Pfeiffer (2013); Pfeiffer et al. (2017); Pfeiffer and Chapman (2019).

17. Pfeiffer and Chapman (2019).

18. Pigg (2001); Biehl (2007).

19. See for example Marks (2002); Zwi and Cabral (1991); Farmer (1992); Nguyen and Peschard (2003); Brodish (2015); Durevall and Lindskog (2012); Ransome et al. (2016); Gillespie (2006); Stillwaggon (2002); Seeley et al. (2012).

20. Crane (2013); Farmer (1999); Mugyenyi (2008); Nguyen (2010).

21. Biehl (2007); Nguyen (2010).

22. The concept of therapeutic economy builds on notions of medical pluralism but emphasizes the link between therapies and wider economic and social relations. See Nguyen (2005); Lock and Nguyen (2010).

23. Cramer (2007, 266; 2001).

24. I build on existing studies of health under neoliberal restructuring, such as Biehl (2005); Benton (2015); Benton, Sangaramoorthy, and Kalofonos (2017); Briggs and Mantini-Briggs (2003); Keshavjee (2014); Sangaramoorthy (2014).

25. Feierman and Janzen (1992)

26. Karp (1997, 394) in Huhn (2016, 181).

27. On personhood in Africa see Radcliffe-Brown (1952); La Fontaine (1985); Fortes (1987); Piot (1991); Englund (1996); Comaroff and Comaroff

(1999); Livingston (2005); Klaits (2010). On personhood outside of Africa see Shweder and Bourne (1982); Markus and Kitayama (1991). Personhood, of course, has a social basis even in the neoliberal West, though this may not be recognized or celebrated.

28. Scherz (2014).

29. Scherz (2014, 2).

30. Miers and Kopytoff (1977); Vansina (1990); Guyer (1993).

31. Ferguson (2013, 226).

32. Feierman (1985).

33. Comaroff (1982, 51).

34. Taussig (1980a).

35. Wendland (2010, 37).

36. In her article examining perspectives on HIV/AIDS among traditional healers in central Mozambique, Bagnol (2017) uses the typology of "natural" and "provoked" or "relational." George Foster proposed a similar typology of "natural" and "personalistic" causes of illness (1976). Green (1996) and Chapman (2010, 192–94) apply Foster's typology to Mozambique.

37. Bagnol (2017).

38. Bourdillon (1982); Chavanduka (1978); Honwana (2002); Lan (1985); Pfeiffer (2002); Bagnol (2017).

39. Honwana (2002); Pfeiffer (2005); Bagnol (2017). There are many types of vengeful spirits outside of the family that often seek to collect a debt contracted by an ancestor as a result of local history. For a discussion of these different types of spirits see Bagnol (2017); Bertelsen (2016).

40. Chapman (2006, 2003); Pfeiffer (2002, 2005); Pfeiffer, Gimbel-Sherr, and Augusto (2007); Bagnol (2017).

41. Bertelsen (2016).

42. Bertelsen (2016).

43. All names of people and local organizations are pseudonyms.

44. Bayart (1993).

45. West (2005, 37).

46. "Bringing rain" and "feeding the people" are references to leaders' roles in providing for their people by appealing to protective spirits to bring rain for the growth of crops. See Ferguson (2006, 73).

47. Auslander (1993); Austen (1993); Comaroff and Comaroff (1999); Geschiere (1997); Mbembe (2001); Parish (2000).

48. Garrido (2012).

49. Ferguson (1990).

50. "Scale-up" has been defined as "an assemblage of vast resources, manpower, expertise, strategies, and technologies, all of which are presumed essential for the implementation of complicated, multifaceted global health interventions throughout and among recipient nations . . . scale-up has become a culture of practice in which new ideological frameworks become dominant and normalized" (Kenworthy and Parker 2014, 2).

51. Foucault (1990); Burchell, Gordon, and Miller (1991).

52. Nguyen (2009, 199); Foucault (1991).

53. Foucault (2003, 254–57); Mbembe (2017, 32–33; 2019, 71).

54. On the submerged forms of race in contemporary development, see Pierre (2020, 95); Kothari (2006); White (2002). On the persistence of colonial ideologies in global health see Greene et al. (2013); Keller (2006); King (2002); Richardson (2019).

55. Holland and Leander define subjectivity as "actors' thoughts, sentiments and embodied sensibilities, and, especially, their sense of self and self-world relations" (2004, 127). Luhrmann adds: "Subjectivity implies the *emotional* experience of a *political* subject, the subject caught up in a world of violence, state authority and pain, the subject's distress under the authority of another" (2006, 346).

56. Rabinow (1992).

57. Mulligan (2017).

58. Petryna (2002, 6).

59. Nguyen (2010, 109).

60. Geographer Matt Sparke (2017) terms this "thin" form biological subcitizenship.

61. Hacking (1986).

62. This expands on the concept of AIDS economy I previously used in Kalofonos (2008, 2010). See also Marsland (2012); Nguyen (2010); Prince (2012, 2014b).

63. Thompson (1971). Political scientist James Scott (1976) popularized the term "moral economy" in analyzing peasant resistance to exploitation by landlords in Southeast Asia.

64. Karandinos et al. (2014); Fassin (2009). The term *moral* in moral economy is not meant to imply that there is something more correct or righteous about systems of norms and obligations that are defined by local worlds of values. Anthropologists use the term to "describe social and historically contingent ethical frameworks that set collective values on specific practices and norms" (Karandinos et al. 2014, 2). Indeed,

anthropologist Philippe Bourgois and colleagues use the concept to make sense of inner-city violence in the United States and to render those acts comprehensible, but not to heroize them (Karandinos et al. 2014). Bourgois and Schonberg use the term to map out the logics of exchange in networks of homeless heroin users (Bourgois 1998; Bourgois and Schonberg 2009). Other anthropologists have used the term to analyze redistributive practices labeled as corruption (Sardan 1999; Smith 2003; Bayart 1993; Bayart, Ellis, and Hibou 1999), the dynamics of witchcraft accusations (Taussig 1986; Austen 1993), and humanitarian medical action (Redfield 2008, 2013). Studying AIDS treatment interventions in West Africa, Vinh-Kim Nguyen uses the term to examine the conflicts that arose when Western "confessional technologies" were brought to West African networks of people living with AIDS, commodifying their testimonials, which had hitherto been used to forge social relationships (Nguyen 2010, 59). Ruth Prince uses the notion of a moral economy in western Kenya to examine the contradictions between the expectations of AIDS treatment programs and material realities (Prince 2012, 537). Moral economy is a tool for thinking about relations of difference and inequality. Highlighting the tensions between distinct moral economies brings attention to what is at stake in contemporary conflicts (Fassin 2009).

65. Fassin (2009, 6); Austen (1993, 92).

66. See Edelman's (2012) critical discussion of the centrality of unequal class relations in Thompson's formulation of the term and his assessment that this aspect has often been lost as the concept has been taken up more broadly in anthropology and the social sciences.

67. See also complementary arguments in Benton (2015); Benton, Sangaramoorthy, and Kalofonos (2017); Braga (2017); and Sangaramoorthy (2014).

68. See Bertelsen's (2016, xv–xvii) detailed discussion of the languages of the region and the many ways ethnicity and language in Central Mozambique have been referred to in the academic literature.

69. Bertelsen (2016); Artur (1999).

70. Bannerman (1993).

71. Bannerman (1993).

72. Artur (1999); Das Neves (1998b).

73. A Portuguese trade magazine reported twenty-five hundred workers were employed when the factory closed (Guerreiro 2003). Text-África CEO Frederico Magalhães told me that more than five thousand

workers were employed at TextÁfrica (personal communication, February 20, 2006).

74. Bertelsen (2016); Das Neves (1998b); Manning (1998); Pitcher (2002). Manning suggests employees of TextÁfrica formed a Renamo "*nucleo*," or cell, during the war.

75. Archambault (2013); Gerety (2018).

76. I analyzed fieldnotes, interview transcripts, and archival documents with qualitative data analysis and extraction software (Text Analysis Markup System Analyzer) that allowed me to thematically code and cross code for keywords and phrases, build charts and concept trees, and systematically compare diverse data. This recursive analysis enabled me to make connections between ethnographic objects and at times produced unexpected results.

CHAPTER 1. POLITICS OF HEALTH AND SURVIVAL

1. See Matsinhe's (2005) use of this metaphor in the title of his excellent account of the early Mozambican response to the HIV/AIDS epidemic. Such a framing also relies on a racialized discourse that positions whiteness and the global north as the source of expert knowledge and the global south as necessarily lacking this (Kothari 2006).

2. The Zimbabwean Plateau refers to an area that encompasses what is today eastern Mozambique and Zimbabwe (Beach 1994, 73–77).

3. Beach (1994, 73).

4. Beach (1980, 24).

5. Newitt (1995, 41–43); Santos (1999).

6. Waite (1992).

7. Isaacman and Isaacman (1983, 37).

8. Allina-Pisano (2002, 25).

9. Ross (1925, 53).

10. Isaacman (1996).

11. Isaacman and Isaacman (1983, 54).

12. Isaacman and Isaacman (1983, 55).

13. Isaacman and Isaacman (1983, 55).

14. Isaacman and Isaacman (1976, 128).

15. Isaacman and Isaacman (1983, 23); Isaacman (1975, 50).

16. Bastos (2007, 767).

17. Shapiro (1983).

18. Prince (2014a). For histories of medicine in Mozambique see Bastos (2007); Dube (2015, 2009); Williams (2013); Honwana (2002, 1996); Shapiro (1983). On colonial responses to indigenous medicine see Feierman (1985); Janzen (1978); Langwick (2011).

19. Honwana (2002, 122–23).

20. Dube (2009); Williams (2013).

21. Mission hospitals were more successful in providing acceptable and effective biomedical care than the Mozambique Company (Dube 2009).

22. Allina (2012, 57).

23. Allina (2012, 58).

24. Feierman (2006); Janzen (1978).

25. Prince (2014a); Feierman (2006).

26. Mamdani (1996); O'Laughlin (2000).

27. Bertelsen (2016, 231–32); O'Laughlin (2000); Penvenne (1995).

28. Beliso-De Jesús and Pierre (2020).

29. Mahoney (2003).

30. Allina (2012); Das Neves (1998b); Isaacman and Sneddon (2000).

31. Mahoney (2003, 173).

32. Reis and Oliveira (2012).

33. Mahoney (2003, 180).

34. West (2005, 151).

35. Newitt (1995, 535–40).

36. Mondlane (1969); Shapiro (1983).

37. Machel quoted in Hanlon (1999, 115).

38. Collins (2006, 9).

39. Collins (2006, 10).

40. Collins (2006, 10).

41. World Bank (1989, 77–78).

42. Mahoney (2003); Machel (1985).

43. This was partly a response to the co-optation by the Portuguese of "traditional" chiefs, called *régulos*, who served as local colonial administrators. See Hanlon (1990), Isaacman and Isaacman (1983), and West (2001, 2005).

44. Newitt (1995, 564).

45. Finnegan (1993, 183).

46. Nordstrom (1998, 104).

47. Finnegan (1993); Nordstrom (1997); Schafer (1998); Roesch (1992); Geffray (1990); Collins (2006).

48. Hanlon (1991, 1).

49. Operation Production (Operação Produção) was an infamous policy that in 1983 forcibly removed urban residents deemed unproductive—defined as prostitutes, vagrants, and traditional and religious authorities—to forced labor and re-education camps in the rural north (Helgesson 1994; Morier-Genoud 1996; Seibert 2005; Vines and Wilson 1995).

50. Brooke (1988).

51. Mondlane (1969).

52. Morier-Genoud (1996).

53. Cruz e Silva (2001b); Das Neves (1998a).

54. Newitt (1995, 436–37).

55. Maxwell (2002).

56. Siegel (2013); Ranger (1987).

57. On the global impact of structural adjustment programs on health see (Pfeiffer and Chapman 2010; Fort et al. 2004; Kim et al. 2000; Kentikelenis, Stubbs, and King 2015; Sparke 2020).

58. Hanlon (1996).

59. Hanlon (1996, 69).

60. The United Nations (1996) defines absolute poverty as "a condition characterized by severe deprivation of basic human needs, including food, safe drinking water, sanitation facilities, health, shelter, education and information. It depends not only on income but also on access to services."

61. Cliff and Noormahomed (1988).

62. Machel (1976); Gloyd, Pfeiffer, and Johnson (2013).

63. See Collins (2006) on the roots of the AIDS epidemic in structural factors shaped by Portuguese colonialism, southern African apartheid regimes, Cold War politics, and structural adjustment. Craddock (2004), Iliffe (2006), and Marks (2002) describe the structural roots of the epidemic in Southern Africa. Iliffe particularly examines why southeastern Africa is the global epicenter of AIDS prevalence and mortality.

64. Hanlon and Smart (2008); Pfeiffer et al. (2017).

65. Pfeiffer (2011).

66. Davis (2004); Pfeiffer (2002); Siegel (2013).

67. Assemblies of God are not PCCs but are a global network, as opposed to the regionally based AICs.

68. Meyer (1998).

69. From a nadir of 75 churches in 1975, the number grew to 456 in March 2000 and 652 in January 2005. The Pentecostal churches (AICs

and PCC) make up the largest percentage of church growth in Mozambique in the postwar period, though these numbers are likely underestimated due to numerous obstacles small churches face to registration (Cruz e Silva 2001a; Seibert 2005). In Chimoio, the Department of Religious Affairs registered over 200 individual AIC and Pentecostal churches in 2002, up from only 30 in the early 1990s. A 2003 survey of three neighborhoods (estimated 1998 population of twenty-one thousand) in Chimoio indicated 45 percent of respondents identified as members of Zionist (25%) or Pentecostal churches (20%), while 23 percent were Catholic (Pfeiffer 2005). Over forty distinctly named church affiliations existed within the Zionist and Pentecostal groups. See Pfeiffer (2003b) on the emergence of a conspicuous culture of international development in central Mozambique.

70. Hanlon (1991).

71. Macamo (2005, 8).

72. Pitcher (2006).

73. World Bank (2007).

74. Hanlon (2007).

75. Hanlon (2007).

76. IMF (2016, 16–17).

77. Mondlane (1969).

78. Cahen (2005).

79. Mavie (2007).

80. White (2002).

81. Hanlon (2009, 3).

82. Rose (1996).

CHAPTER 2. THE EMERGENCE OF THE AIDS ECONOMY

1. Prince (2012, 2016); Whyte (2014); Benton (2015); Nguyen (2010); Benton, Sangaramoorthy, and Kalofonos (2017).

2. Nguyen (2005, 126).

3. West (2005, 46).

4. Healers and nonhealers alike commonly compared HIV/AIDS to both *piringaniso* and *tsanganiko*, both resulting from a failure to observe social rules around sexuality, death, and burial. See a nuanced account of these diseases in Bagnol (2017).

5. Bagnol (2017); Niehaus (2007).

6. See the detailed discussion of various theories along these lines in Bagnol (2017).

7. On the complexities of this history, see Bertelsen (2016), West (2005), Meneses (2007), and Honwana (1996, 2002). In postliberation Mozambique, modernization's goal was "not only the eradication of underdevelopment, but also the creation of a socialist society based on a workers-peasants alliance and . . . aimed at creating a 'new man', i.e. one emancipated from the oppressive weight of tradition" (Macamo and Neubert 2004: 65; see also Farré 2015.

8. Pfeiffer (2004a).

9. Taussig (1980b, 117).

10. Farmer (1992); Ashforth (2010).

11. In *The Quest for Therapy in Lower Zaire*, Janzen (1978) famously wrote about "therapy managing groups" that debate options and make decisions about which practitioners to consult and when on economic and cultural grounds.

12. For more on *capulanas* see Arnfred and Meneses (2018).

13. Chapman (2010).

14. Bourdillon (1982).

15. Pfeiffer (2003a).

16. Pfeiffer, Gimbel-Sherr, and Augusto (2007); Pfeiffer (2002, 2005).

17. Whyte (2002, 172).

18. Matsinhe (2005, 80); Høg (2008). This fear-based strategy was globally circulating in an atmosphere of panic as the world grappled with the implications of an emerging epidemic that seemed to have few effective responses (Seidel 1993).

19. See a description and picture of this poster in Matsinhe (2005, 83).

20. Treichler (1999); Setel (1999); Farmer (1992); Matsinhe (2005).

21. Ashforth (2010); Niehaus (2007).

22. Agadjanian (2002, 208).

23. Individuals were more willing to disclose if there was payment involved. See Nguyen (2010) on the corrosive effects this commodification of testimonials around HIV/AIDS interventions had in West African settings of precarity, leading to competition, suspicion, and fractured solidarities.

24. Gluckman (1956).

25. Austen (1993); Newell (2007).

26. Newell (2007, 462).

27. Dilger (2012).

28. Nguyen (2010, ch. 1).

29. Nguyen (2010).

30. Seidel (1993).

31 In the early years of the epidemic in the United States, HIV cases initially surfaced among "the four H's:" Haitians, injection drug (heroin) users, recipients of blood products (hemophiliacs), and homosexuals. See Crimp (1988), Patton (1990), and Treichler (1999).

32. Epstein (1996).

33. See Morolake, Stephens, and Welbourn (2009) for an overview of GIPA. Nguyen critiques GIPA for being tied to a model of self-help that assumes the existence of a "hidden truth to the self" that must be shared in order to achieve personal catharsis and form social bonds, an assumption that does not fit with African contexts where social bonds are often formed through networks of obligation, responsibility and exchange that do not require self-disclosure (2010, 83). Anthropologist Adia Benton argues GIPA reduces involvement by people living with HIV/AIDS to public visibility, thus reducing opportunities to be involved without one's serostatus being made public (2015, 92–93).

34. Dilger (2001); Whyte (1997).

35. Harrington (2008). See also the discussion on the roots of positive living in Africa in Benton, Sangaramoorthy, and Kalofonos (2017).

36. Orr (2003).

37. Orr (2003).

38. Orr (2003, 88).

39. The African potato is a medicinal plant in southern Africa that was rumored to be beneficial for people with HIV/AIDS prior to the ARV scale-up (Drewes and Khan 2004).

40. Matsinhe (2005, 60).

41. Conselho Nacional De Combate Ao HIV/SIDA (2004).

42. Foucault (2008, 226); Dumont (1977).

43. Prince (2012, 535).

44. Macamo (2006).

45. Macamo (2006).

46. Epstein (2007, 83).

47. Setel (1999); Smith (2014).

48. Pfeiffer (2003b, 2004b).

49. Nguyen (2010, 109).

50. Nguyen (2010, 176–78).

51. Ferguson (2006, 85).

52. Kothari (2006, 15). See also Pierre (2020).

53. Alongside witchcraft, the figure of the zombie is used throughout sub-Saharan Africa to refer to alienated labor power, abducted from the home in order to serve as someone else's instrument of production. The figure of the zombie has clear resonances with slavery. See Comaroff and Comaroff (2012) and Geschiere (1997).

54. Fassin (2009, 11).

55. Scott (1976) in Fassin (2009, 11).

56. Comaroff (1985, 225); Luedke (2007, 722).

CHAPTER 3. THERAPEUTIC CONGREGATIONS

1. Iliffe (2006).

2. Dilger (2001).

3. This chapter and the next draw on the literature on healing and Christianity in contemporary Mozambique and Africa in general (see, for example, Livingston 2012; Honwana 2002; Pfeiffer 2002; Dilger 2007). Erica Bornstein (2005) has written about the intersection of contemporary forms of Christianity with international development, and there is literature examining the intersection of Christianity and HIV/AIDS interventions (Becker and Geissler 2009; Van dijk et al. 2014; Burchardt 2015; Prince, Denis, and Van dijk 2009).

4. IMF (2016).

5. Chapman (2010, 185).

6. See also Dilger's (2010) detailed case studies of families caring for loved ones suffering from AIDS in Tanzania that show how the meanings and practices surrounding families' struggles over illness, death, and survival and the fatigue of caregivers are embedded in regional political economies of health care as well as in social and cultural processes through which moral and familial belonging as well as the past and the future are all negotiated.

7. Scheper-Hughes (1992, 405).

8. Meyer (1998).

9. The CD4 count is a test measuring the blood serum concentration of an immune cell that HIV attacks. The CD4 count was clinically used as an indicator of the health of the immune system and to assess how well antiretroviral treatment was working. See chapter 5 for more discussion of the CD4 count and how it was mobilized in *Vida Positiva* and counseling discourses as a moral barometer reflecting proper self-care.

10. Ashforth (2010); Niehaus (2007).

11. Brandt and Rozin (1997); Iliffe (2006).

12. See Meyer (1998). Many who "lived positively" decried the time and money they wasted with *n'angas* and *profetas* but nevertheless might still seek them out under the right circumstances, partly because it was not always completely up to the sick individual, but rather members of the social network who influenced which therapies were pursued.

13. Bertelsen (2016).

14. Hardiman (2006).

15. Arnfred (2004).

16. Burchardt (2015, 169).

17. Macamo (2005).

18. Whyte (1997, 223).

19. NDPB (2004).

20. See Nguyen (2010) for similar accounts of schism in associations of people living with HIV/AIDS in West Africa.

21. Lisa Richey (2011) discusses a similar predicament HIV positive women faced in South African AIDS clinics.

22. Chapman (2010, 167).

23. Infertility was a commonly cited reason for divorce in contemporary Chimoio. Historically for the Shona, the main purpose of marriage was the continuation and growth of the family group (Bourdillon 1982). The wife traditionally received her cooking stones, symbolic of the marriage, only after the birth of the first child. Infertility on the part of the wife, whether inability to get pregnant or frequent miscarriage, was regarded as failure by the wife's family to fulfill their side of the marriage contract, necessitating provision of another daughter or return of the bride-price, *lobolo*. The payment of *lobolo* extends over a long period, often a lifetime, as the husband ensures his wife bears him a number of children for his lineage. The wife's family also can demand favors in the form of service or gifts as long as the son-in-law remains indebted to them (Chapman 2010, 161–62; Bourdillon 1982). Parenthood is thus important to establish adult status, to consolidate a marriage, and for the wife to secure her own status in the husband's home.

24. Fassin (2007); Hunter (2010).

25. In the postsocialist, neoliberal era, there has been an effort to revitalize institutions of traditional authority as efficient and effective mechanisms of local authority that provide residents with a means to manage their own affairs at no cost to the state. Northern donors have played a significant

role in advancing this vision, which relies on a simplistic and romanticized idea of "tradition" (West 2005; Buur and Kyed 2006; Obarrio 2015).

26. Prince (2007, 89).

27. Ferguson (2006); Pigg (1996); Whyte (2002).

28. Culturalism amounts to a pathologization of culture and leads to blaming the victims of structural violence for higher rates of disease and their restricted health-care options (Farmer 1999; Fassin 2001; Lock and Nguyen 2010; Briggs and Mantini-Briggs 2003). For historical perspectives, see Vaughan (1991) and Ranger (1981).

29. Nguyen (2005, 2010); Nguyen et al. (2007).

30. Bourgois (2005); Bourgois and Schonberg (2009).

31. Beste and Pfeiffer (2016).

32. Cunguara and Hanlon (2010).

CHAPTER 4. THE USES OF COMMUNITY LABOR

1. TASO, the Ugandan organization that pioneered positive living and associations of people living with HIV/AIDS, is also one of the earliest and most frequently cited African models of CHBC. TASO activists worked with hospital staff to train and support family members caring for people with HIV/AIDS at home starting in the late 1980s (Iliffe 2006, 106).

2. UNAIDS (2002, 2010).

3. Simone (2004).

4. Maes (2012).

5. Kleinman and Hanna (2008).

6. Ferguson (2006); Prince (2014b); Sullivan (2011); Wendland (2012).

7. The other initiatives, pastor and youth education and training for HIV/AIDS prevention, are not discussed here.

8. As elsewhere, volunteers visited all suffering from chronic disease in order to avoid visiting only people with HIV/AIDS and thereby inadvertently revealing someone's serostatus.

9. Prince (2014b).

10. See, for example, Muchano (2006).

11. See Maes (2012) for an example of similar dynamic in Ethiopia with a secular organization and Maes and Kalofonos (2013) and Maes, Closser, and Kalofonos (2014) for comparisons across countries.

12. Janzen (1978).

13. Janzen (1978).

14. Newell (2006, 180). While *n'angas* and *profetes* had standardized payment charts created by AMETRAMO specifying the official charges for various services, in Arminda's father's time, payment was more often informal and in-kind, consisting of gifts of produce, livestock, or labor. Many healers still accepted these forms of payment.

15. Honwana (2002); Meyer (2004); Pfeiffer (2002).

16. Community-based care volunteers and community health workers more broadly can be seen to express these motivations in contexts across Africa (Akintola 2011; Maes and Kalofonos 2013; Maes 2012; Prince 2015; Rödlach 2009; Swidler and Watkins 2009).

17. PNCS (2004, 43).

18. PNCS (2004, 43).

19. The "community and other social sectors" are also referenced, but the majority of new services were biomedical.

20. This emphasis on data collection, monitoring, and surveillance is a part of the rise of "audit culture" in global health that is characterized by "managers and accountants usurping the role of actual experts in evaluating and measuring performance" (Pfeiffer 2019, 52). Audit culture is a part of neoliberal logics of austerity, privatization, downsizing, outsourcing, and decentralization that serves to infuse health with the logic of economics (Adams 2016; Strathern 2000; Shore and Wright 1997).

21. Arthur Kleinman explores the degradation of the ethics of care in contemporary biomedicine as technological and financial considerations drive practice. See for example Kleinman (2015, 2012), Kleinman and Hanna (2008), and Kleinman (1995).

22. This can be seen as part of a broader audit culture in global health partnerships entailing the proliferation of documentation practices (McKay 2018, 2012; Shore and Wright 1997; Strathern 2000; Pfeiffer 2019; Gimbel et al. 2018).

23. Swartz (2013) similarly discusses distinct experiences along generational lines for CHWs in South Africa.

24. The pace and scale of Mufudzi's growth was not atypical of the trajectory of similar organizations across Africa at the time. See Droggitis and Oomman (2010) and Oomman, Bernstein, and Rosenzweig (2007).

25. MISAU (2006, 10).

26. See Sherr et al. (2012) for a discussion on the dynamic of internal brain drain from the public health sector to donor agencies, NGOs, and the private sector.

27. These amounts were down from the 2006 allotment of 36 kg rice, 18 kg CSB, 6kg legumes, and 1.5 L oil. The available food supplements did not keep pace with increasing numbers of patients.

28. See discussions on the social and emotional impacts of unpaid volunteer work in Ethiopia in Maes and Shifferaw (2011) and Maes (2016).

29. Hanlon and Smart (2008); Pfeiffer (2003a).

30. Pfeiffer and Chapman (2010).

31. Prince (2015).

32. Swartz (2013, 140).

33. Lehmann and Sanders (2007).

34. Ferguson (2006).

35. Sullivan (2011); Wendland (2012).

36. Gershon (2011, 537); Foucault (2008).

37. Allan (2019); Kuehn and Corrigan (2013).

38. Ferguson (2013, 2015).

39. Prince (2015).

CHAPTER 5. BEING SEEN IN THE DAY HOSPITAL

1. Cliff (1993); Hanlon (1996).

2. Gloyd (1996).

3. *Técnicos de medicina* have two and a half to three years of training compared to six for physicians.

4. This phrase is from Harries et al. (2001). See also Stevens, Kaye, and Corrah (2004).

5. Anthropologists Eileen Moyer and Anita Hardon (2014) discuss the tensions between normalization and exceptionalism of HIV/AIDS in their introduction to a special issue of *Medical Anthropology* entitled "The Normalization of HIV in the Age of Antriretroviral Treatment: Perspectives from Everyday Practice." See also Benton's (2015) ethnography of the unanticipated consequences of HIV exceptionalism in the comparatively low-prevalence African setting of Sierra Leone (2015).

6. De Maeseneer et al. (2008); England (2007).

7. Høg (2014); Sontag, LaFraniere, and Wines (2004).

8. Pfeiffer (2013). The "vertical" approach goes along with neoliberal assumptions of limited resources for health and a private sector, business mentality to health care that foregrounds concepts such as "cost effectiveness," "return on investment," "results-based management," and "performance-based financing" (Pfeiffer 2019).

9. Høg (2014); Oomman, Bernstein, and Rosenzweig (2007).

10. On the creation of high-tech enclaves by global health, see Sparke (2014); Wendland (2012); Sullivan (2011).

11. The Integrated Health Network model is laid out in Conselho Nacional De Combate Ao HIV/SIDA (2004). This model changed in 2008 when the Day Hospitals closed and AIDS care was integrated into the general primary care clinics. This chapter focuses on the care provided in the Day Hospitals between 2004 and 2006.

12. See anthropologist Ramah McKay's (2012, 2018) insightful analysis of the role proliferating documentation from multiple authorities played in complicating care in an AIDS clinic in Maputo. This is a part of the growing audit culture in global health (Pfeiffer 2019; Adams 2016; Strathern 2000; Shore and Wright 1997; Gimbel et al. 2018).

13. Unlike CHBC volunteers discussed in the previous chapter, *agentes terapêuticos* had to have a minimum level of secondary education and were expected to be literate in Portuguese. In keeping with a national and global political economy that valued technically oriented work above forms of care deemed "social" and "emotional," *agentes terapêuticos* were compensated from the start. Their positions were created in the early 2000s, at the start of the treatment scale-up, while CHBC was begun in the mid-1990s, prior to the treatment scale-up.

14. Cliff (1991); Hanlon (1999); Lubkemann (2001).

15. Patients who were symptomatic on their first visit would be triaged by nurses and if necessary see a doctor or the medical assistant that day for acute care. If not, they had a follow-up visit to have their CD4 count read in two weeks. If the CD4 count was above 200 and the patient was asymptomatic, they did not meet biological criteria for treatment and would be scheduled to return for another CD4 count in six months. They met biological criteria if the CD4 count was less than 200, or less than 350 with certain clinical criteria, or they had clinical signs of advanced AIDS regardless of CD4 count. In these cases, they were referred for an appointment with a physician and a social worker (PNCS 2004). These were the standard global criteria for treatment at the time, but they contrast with current guidelines for all HIV positive adults to begin treatment regardless of CD4 count or clinical disease.

16. This would later be modified to visits every two weeks for two months.

17. Whyte et al. (2013, 164).

18. Ferguson (2015).

19. "Socialization for scarcity" was the title of a study on child feeding practices in Haiti (Alvarez and Murray 1981). The term has been popularized by Paul Farmer to emphasize the fact that scarcity is often a policy choice, not a reflection of available resources (Farmer 1988, 2004; Farmer et al. 2013)

20. O'Laughlin (1996).

21. The term *moral barometer* was used by Farmer: "Bad blood and spoiled milk serve as moral barometers that submit 'private' problems (abuse of women, especially pregnant or nursing ones) to public scrutiny" (1988, 62). In this case, CD4 counts submitted private behavior to clinical scrutiny.

22. Crane (2013, 44).

23. A US study found ARV drug resistance to be the most concentrated among highly adherent patients rather than those who frequently missed doses. Patients with the worst adherence (under 65 percent) had little drug resistance as well as little clinical benefit from the treatment. These researchers argued the relationship between poor adherence and drug resistance was different for different types of ARVs. Older classes of ARVs seemed to be more susceptible to the development of resistance in response to missed doses than the newer classes, such as the protease inhibitor drugs. Unfortunately, it was the older classes of ARVs that were generically produced and were thus the cheapest and most widely available option in Africa (Cipla's Triomune). Despite the anxieties in the global north about resistance as a public health problem, the ARVs that were provided to Africa were those that were the least expensive and the most likely to cause resistance if doses were missed (Bangsberg et al. 2003; Bangsberg, Moss, and Deeks 2004; Crane 2013, ch. 1).

24. Seeley et al. (2012).

25. Crane (2013, 35); Messac and Prabhu (2013, 115–19). The term *unsanitary subjects* is from Briggs and Mantini-Briggs (2003, 10).

26. Crane (2013, 36); Briggs and Mantini-Briggs (2003, xvi).

27. Gusdal et al. (2009); Lubega et al. (2010).

28. Messac and Prabhu (2013); Farmer et al. (2001); MSF Africa (2003).

29. Crane (2013, 38).

30. Anthropologist Carla Braga discusses a similar dynamic in AIDS treatment in Chimoio from 2007 to 2013. She argues that in practice, the conception of modernity continues to be associated with an urban way of life, tidiness, education, and the ability to speak Portuguese, and these factors "constitute the grid on the basis of which health workers

take decisions" (2017, 239). This chapter's argument, that poor Mozambi-cans had to earn access to ARVs by proving their ability to live positively and adhere to medications, complements Braga's argument that health workers gave preferential treatment to patients embodying conceptions of modernity.

31. Farmer (1999, 9).

32. SETSAN (2008).

33. Weiser et al. (2011).

34. *Hearing on the United States' War on AIDS* (2001).

35. See note 23 in this chapter.

36. Cruikshank (1993, 328).

37. Ferguson and Gupta (2002).

38. Elisha (2008).

39. Mukherjee (2000).

40. Crane (2013, 34).

41. Mussa et al. (2013); Sherr et al. (2012).

42. Lambdin et al. (2013) present the justification of the integration of AIDS treatment into the broader primary health system, which is sound from the perspective of systems equity. Yet their study indicates a higher dropout rate in the integrated programs than in the vertical, Day Hospi-tal model.

43. Braga (2012); Olsen (2013); Reed (2014, 2018).

CHAPTER 6. HUNGER AS EMBODIED CRITIQUE

1. Scheper-Hughes (1992, 135).

2. Scheper-Hughes (1993, 221); Scheper-Hughes and Lock (1987).

3. Bayart (1993).

4. Shevitz (1999).

5. Serwadda et al. (1985).

6. Stillwaggon (2006, 2002).

7. De Waal and Whiteside (2003). Also see Gillespie (2006).

8. Phiri (2012).

9. SETSAN (2008).

10. NDPB (2004).

11. Weiser et al (2011) provide a comprehensive review of all the ways food insecurity can lead to both increased HIV transmission between people as well as disease progression in an individual, including: macro and micronutrient deficiencies that can lead to increased HIV

transmission, immunologic decline and increased morbidity and mortality in those infected; increased depression and drug abuse which can contribute to HIV transmission risk, incomplete HIV viral load suppression, and increased morbidity and mortality among HIV-infected individuals; enhanced HIV transmission through direct attempts to procure food, such as transactional or "survival" sex; antiretroviral therapy nonadherence, treatment interruptions, and missed clinic visits.

12. See critiques of sustainability in Farmer (1999); Swidler and Watkins (2009); Ferguson (2015).

13. Minutes from Working Group on Nutrition and ART, March 28, 2005.

14. Initially, need was subjectively defined by the Day Hospital staff. Later need was defined in terms of anthropometric criteria including Body Mass Index and upper arm circumference.

15. This slang term comes from the American television series titled "MacGyver" that aired in North America from 1985 to 1992, and featured a resourceful secret agent who improvised complex devices out of improbable household materials to solve apparently intractable problems. The program aired on local television, and was popular in *bairro* cinemas—structures of bamboo and tarp where a television was set up. "*Magaiva*" and "*James Bond*" referred to clever actors who devised schemes for resource acquisition, seemingly against all odds, and often through illicit means.

16. Bertelsen (2016); Kyed (2007).

17. Scherz (2014); Ferguson (2013, 2015).

18. Mavie (2007); Agência Moçambicana de Informação (2007).

19. Ferguson (2013).

20. On Xiconhoca, see Isaacman and Isaacman (1983); Macamo (2017, 2005); Meneses (2015).

21. *Notícias* (2006).

22. Oomman, Bernstein, and Rosenzweig (2008, 2007) (majority of funds); Costello (2008) (pharmaceutical firms' profits).

23. Pfeiffer et al. (2017).

24. Bond (2007); Høg (2014).

25. Hunt cited in Crane (2013, 169). Crane uses Hunt's observation to question whether contemporary global health interventions reproduce these historical dynamics in terms of the extraction of scientific data and the creation of sites for research and experimentation and enacting forms of salvation through dramatic biomedical cures, such as AIDS treatment.

26. Keshavjee (2014).

27. Dubal (2018); Englund (2006); Fassin (2012); Prince (2012); Ticktin (2011).

28. Sparke (2020); Glasgow and Schrecker (2016).

29. Whyte (2014, 207).

30. Bertelsen (2016); Huhn (2016); West (2005).

31. Kleinman (1995, 35).

32. Farmer (1999); Dubal (2012, 2018).

33. Birn and Richter (2018).

34. Rees (2014).

35. This paraphrases Nguyen (2010, 182). See also Petryna (2002); Kalofonos (2019).

36. The term philanthrocapitalism refers to "both infusing philanthropy with the principles and practices of for-profit enterprise and as a way of demonstrating capitalism's benevolent potential through innovations that allegedly 'benefit everyone, sooner or later, through new products, higher quality, and lower prices'" (Birn and Richter 2018, 157).

37. Birn and Richter (2018); Giridharadas (2018).

38. Brandt (2013).

39. Gray (2013); Epstein (1996); Grebe (2011); Messac and Prabhu (2013); D'Adesky (2006) (potential to shift policy). The HIV/AIDS epidemic continues to exact a devastating toll not only in sub-Saharan Africa, but in under-resourced socially precarious communities globally, particularly in LGBTQ communities of color (Villarosa 2017; Wilson, Wright, and Isbell 2008; Sangaramoorthy 2014, 2018).

40. Birn and Richter (2018).

41. Horton (2018).

42. Metzl and Hansen (2014); Holmes, Greene, and Stonington (2014); Stonington et al. (2018); Bourgois et al. (2017); Dubal (2018).

43. Taylor and Rieger (1984); Waitzkin (2006) (re: Virchow). This is Horton's argument in his 2018 *Lancet* editorial (Fanon 1967, 1961, 1965).

44. Werner, Thuman, and Maxwell (2017) ("Where There Is No Doctor"); Maes (2016) ("Where There Is No Labor Movement").

45. Pfeiffer (2013).

46. The code calls for foreign NGOs to avoid luring local staff of public-sector health systems to their projects, to support local Ministry of Health priority setting, to avoid creation of parallel systems, and to advocate for debt relief and increases in public-sector spending (Pfeiffer et al. 2008). On the daunting challenges faced by the sector wide approach see Pfeiffer et al. (2017) and Sparke (2020).

47. Pfeiffer and Chapman (2019).

48. See the special issue "The Political Determinants of Health Inequities and Universal Health Coverage," *Globalization and Health* Supp. 1 (2019), particularly Birn and Nervi (2019) on the history and politics of current efforts to move towards universal health coverage on a global scale.

49. Epidemiologists Kate Pickett and Richard Wilkinson (2010) demonstrate that inequality is correlated with a host of health and social problems.

50. The hunger of patients on ARVs has never been systematically addressed in national AIDS treatment programs. A food voucher program for people on ARVs has been piloted and sporadically implemented with some reports of success (Pfeiffer 2013; Umberg 2015). The voucher program addressed the logistical complexities, but not the issue of triage, as the food voucher was still granted for a limited time according to specific criteria for a limited number of people. Integrated HIV and livelihood programs have been proposed to target the root causes of food insecurity (Yager, Kadiyala, and Weiser 2011; Weiser et al. 2015). These typically support clients in small-enterprise, crop production and animal husbandry, provide productive skills and capital, bolstering livelihood and not just providing food (Kadiyala et al. 2009). Some of the associations and groups I encountered in Mozambique were engaging in these types of activities and they were eagerly endorsed by those lucky enough to be in them, when their illness allowed it.

51. Feinglass, Gomes, and Maru (2016).

52. Audet et al. (2015).

53. Jobarteh et al. (2016).

54. James Scott points out the downfalls of an "imperial or hegemonic planning mentality that excludes the necessary role of local knowledge and know-how" regardless of political ideology (1998, 6).

55. Ferguson points to the growing interest in southern Africa and across the globe in redistributive policies that replace tattered social safety nets, at best designed to catch only those who "fall," with a social protection floor, "a universal citizenship right that provides all with some minimal place to stand" (2015, 211). A social protection floor would include universal health coverage with investment in health infrastructure as well as attention to livelihood in the form of universal large-scale cash transfer programs. These programs provide a minimum basic income and standard of living to all and have been shown to alleviate poverty and stimulate local economies (Hanlon, Barrientos, and Hulme 2010). They are an effort

to build an inclusive economy in which all can rely on having access to the basic minimum.

56. International Labour Organization (2012).

57. Hanlon, Barrientos, and Hulme (2010).

58. Ruckert and Labonté (2017).

59. Achiume (2019); Williams and Collins (2004).

60. Auld et al. (2016); Lambdin et al. (2013).

61. Brito et al. (2014).

62. See Joseph Hanlon's (2020a) analysis of the armed uprising in Cabo Delgado. This uprising occurs while the government has agreed to $5.7 billion worth of loans that are estimated to result in nearly 30,000 jobs for US and UK citizens and less than 2500 for Mozambicans (Hanlon 2020b).

63. Boerner (2020); Kelley et al. (2020); Shamasunder et al. (2020).

64. Lancet Editorial (2020); Associated Press (2020).

65. World Health Organization (2020); UNAIDS (2020).

References

Achiume, Tendayi. 2019. *Report of the Special Rapporteur on Contemporary Forms of Racism, Racial Discrimination, Xenophobia and Racial Intolerance.* Geneva: United Nations General Assembly.

Adams, Vincanne. 2016. *Metrics: What Counts in Global Health.* Durham, NC: Duke University Press. https://doi.org/10.1515/9780822374480.

Agadjanian, Victor. 2002. "Informal Social Networks and Epidemic Prevention in a Third World Context: Cholera and HIV/AIDS Compared." In *Social Networks and Health*, edited by Judith A. Levy and Bernice A. Pescosolido, 201–21. West Yorkshire, UK: Emerald Group Publishing Limited. https://doi.org/10.1016/S1057-6290(02)80027-4.

Agéncia Moçambicana de Informação. 2007. *Guebuza diz que adultos não podem eesperar como crianças.* December 10.

Akintola, Olagoke. 2011. "What Motivates People to Volunteer? The Case of Volunteer AIDS Caregivers in Faith-Based Organizations in KwaZulu-Natal, South Africa." *Health Policy and Planning* 26 (1): 53–62. https://doi.org/10.1093/heapol/czq019.

Allan, Kori. 2019. "Volunteering as Hope Labour: The Potential Value of Unpaid Work Experience for the Un- and Under-Employed." *Culture,*

Theory and Critique 60 (1): 66–83. https://doi.org/10.1080/14735784
.2018.1548300.

Allina, Eric. 2012. *Slavery by Any Other Name: African Life under Company Rule in Colonial Mozambique*. Charlottesville: University of Virginia Press.

Allina-Pisano, Eric. 2002. "Negotiating Colonialism: Africans, the State, and the Market in Manica District, Mozambique 1895–c. 1935." PhD diss., Yale University.

Alvarez, Maria, and Gerald Murray. 1981. *Socialization for Scarcity: Child Feeding Beliefs and Practices in a Haitian Village*. Port-au-Prince: USAID.

Archambault, Julie Soleil. 2013. "Cruising through Uncertainty: Cell Phones and the Politics of Display and Disguise in Inhambane, Mozambique." *American Ethnologist* 40 (1): 88–101. https://doi.org/10.1111/amet.12007.

Arnfred, Signe. 2004. "Conceptions of Gender in Colonial and Post-Colonial Discourses: The Case of Mozambique." In *Gender Activism and Studies in Africa*, edited by CODESRIA, 108–28. Dakar: CODESRIA.

Arnfred, Signe, and Maria Paula Meneses. 2018. "Mozambican Capulanas: Tracing Histories and Memories." In *Mozambique on the Move*, edited by Sheila Pereira Khan, Maria Paula Meneses, and Bjørn Enge Bertelsen, 186–210. Leiden: Brill. https://doi.org/10.1163/9789004381100_011.

Artur, Domingos do Rosário. 1999. *Cidade de Chimoio: Ensaio histórico-sociológico*. Edited by Luís Covane. Colecção Embondeiro, 14. Chimoio, Mozambique: ARPAC.

Ashforth, Adam. 2010. "Spiritual Insecurity and AIDS in South Africa." In *Morality, Hope, and Grief: Anthropologies of AIDS in Africa*, edited by Hansjörg Dilger and Ute Luig, 43–60. New York: Berghahn Books.

Associated Press. 2020. "Sex Workers in Africa Lack Food for Taking HIV Drugs during Coronavirus Outbreak." *Los Angeles Times*, July 4. www.latimes.com/world-nation/story/2020-07-04/sex-workers-lack-food-for-taking-hiv-drugs-during-covid-19.

Audet, Carolyn M., Erin Hamilton, Leighann Hughart, and Jose Salato. 2015. "Engagement of Traditional Healers and Birth Attendants as a Controversial Proposal to Extend the HIV Health Workforce." *Current HIV/AIDS Reports* 12 (2): 238–45. https://doi.org/10.1007/s11904-015-0258-8.

Auld, Andrew F., Ray W. Shiraishi, Aleny Couto, Francisco Mbofana, Kathryn Colborn, Charity Alfredo, Tedd V. Ellerbrock, Carla Xavier, and Kebba Jobarteh. 2016. "A Decade of Antiretroviral Therapy Scale-up in Mozambique: Evaluation of Outcome Trends and New Models of Service Delivery among More Than 300,000 Patients Enrolled during 2004–2013." *Journal of Acquired Immune Deficiency Syndromes* 73 (2): 11–22. https://doi.org/10.1097/QAI.0000000000001137.

Auslander, Mark. 1993. "'Open the Wombs!': The Symbolic Politics of Modern Ngoni Witchfinding." In *Modernity and Its Malcontents: Ritual and Power in Postcolonial Africa*, edited by Jean Comaroff and John L. Comaroff, 167–92. Chicago: University of Chicago Press.

Austen, Ralph A. 1993. "The Moral Economy of Witchcraft: An Essay in Comparative History." In *Modernity and Its Malcontents : Ritual and Power in Postcolonial Africa*, edited by Jean Comaroff and John L. Comaroff, 89–110. Chicago: University of Chicago Press.

Bagnol, Brigitte. 2017. "The Aetiology of Diseases in Central Mozambique: With a Special Focus on HIV/AIDS." *African Studies* 76 (2): 205–20. https://doi.org/10.1080/00020184.2017.1322867.

Bangsberg, David R., Edwin D. Charlebois, Robert M. Grant, Mark Holodniy, Steven G. Deeks, Sharon Perry, Kathleen Nugent Conroy, et al. 2003. "High Levels of Adherence Do Not Prevent Accumulation of HIV Drug Resistance Mutations." *AIDS* 17: 1925–32.http//doi.org/10.1097/01.aids.0000076320.42412.fd.

Bangsberg, David R., Andrew R. Moss, and Steven G. Deeks. 2004. "Paradoxes of Adherence and Drug Resistance to HIV Antiretroviral Therapy." *Journal of Antimicrobial Chemotherapy* 53 (5): 696–99. https://doi.org/10.1093/jac/dkh162.

Bannerman, John H. 1993. *Land Tenure Past and Present in the Manica Province of Moçambique*. Chimoio: Report prepared for Mozambique Agricultural Rural Construction Programme (MAARP), supported by the German Agency for Technical Cooperation (GTZ).

Bastos, Cristiana. 2007. "Medical Hybridisms and Social Boundaries: Aspects of Portuguese Colonialism in Africa and India in the Nineteenth Century." *Journal of Southern African Studies* 33 (4): 767–82. https://doi.org/10.1080/03057070701646878.

Bayart, Jean-François. 1993. *The State in Africa: The Politics of the Belly*. London: Longman.

Bayart, Jean-François, Stephen Ellis, and Béatrice Hibou. 1999. *The Criminalization of the State in Africa*. Bloomington: Indiana University Press.

Beach, D. N. 1980. *The Shona and Zimbabwe, 900–1850: An Outline of Shona History*. Zambeziana, vol. 9. Gwelo: Mambo.

———. 1994. *The Shona and Their Neighbours. The Peoples of Africa*. Cambridge, MA: Blackwell.

Becker, Felicitas, and P. W. Geissler. 2009. *AIDS and Religious Practice in Africa*. Leiden: Brill.

Beliso-De Jesús, Aisha M., and Jemima Pierre. 2020. "Special Section: Anthropology of White Supremacy." *American Anthropologist* 122 (1): 65–75. https://doi.org/10.1111/aman.13351.

Benton, Adia. 2015. *HIV Exceptionalism: Development through Disease in Sierra Leone*. Minneapolis: University of Minnesota Press.

Benton, Adia, Thurka Sangaramoorthy, and Ippolytos Kalofonos. 2017. "Temporality and Positive Living in the Age of HIV/AIDS: A Multi-sited Ethnography." *Current Anthropology* 58 (4): 454–76. https://doi.org/10.1086/692825.

Bertelsen, Bjørn Enge. 2016. *Violent Becomings: State Formation, Sociality and Power in Mozambique*. New York: Berghahn Books.

Beste, Jason, and James Pfeiffer. 2016. "Mozambique's Debt and the International Monetary Fund's Influence on Poverty, Education, and Health." *International Journal of Health Services* 46 (2): 366–81. https://doi.org/10.1177/0020731416637062.

Biehl, João. 2005. *Vita: Life in a Zone of Social Abandonment*. Berkeley: University of California Press.

———. 2007. *Will to Live: AIDS Therapies and the Politics of Survival*. Princeton, NJ: Princeton University Press.

Birn, Anne-Emanuelle, and Laura Nervi. 2019. "What Matters in Health (Care) Universes: Delusions, Dilutions, and Ways towards Universal Health Justice." *Globalization and Health* 15 (Supp. 1): 1–12. https://doi.org/10.1186/s12992-019-0521-7.

Birn, Anne-Emanuelle, and Judith Richter. 2018. "U.S. Philanthrocapitalism and the Global Health Agenda—PEAH—Policies for Equitable Access to Health." In *Health Care under the Knife: Moving Beyond Capitalism for Our Health*, edited by Howard Waitzkin and Working Group on Health Beyond Capitalism, 155–74. New York: Monthly Review Press.

Boerner, Heather. 2020. "Lessons from the HIV Epidemic for the COVID-19 Pandemic." Medscape. www.medscape.com/viewarticle/928300.

Bond, Patrick. 2007. "The Dispossession of African Wealth at the Cost of Africa's Health." *International Journal of Health Services* 37 (1): 171–92. https://doi.org/10.2190/UK65-4235-N866-3R34.

Bornstein, Erica. 2005. *The Spirit of Development: Protestant NGOs, Morality, and Economics in Zimbabwe*. Stanford, CA: Stanford University Press.

Bourdillon, M. F. C. 1982. *The Shona Peoples: An Ethnography of the Contemporary Shona, with Special Reference to Their Religion*. Gweru, Zimbabwe: Mambo Press.

Bourgois, Philippe. 1998. "The Moral Economies of Homeless Heroin Addicts: Confronting Ethnography, HIV Risk, and Everyday Violence in San Francisco Shooting Encampments." *Substance Use and Misuse* 33 (11): 2323–51. https://doi.org/10.3109/10826089809056260.

———. 2005. "Missing the Holocaust: My Father's Account of Auschwitz from August 1943 to June 1944." *Anthropological Theory* 78 (1): 89–123.

Bourgois, Philippe, Seth M. Holmes, Kimberly Lauren Sue, and James Quesada. 2017. "Structural Vulnerability: Operationalizing the Concept to Address Health Disparities in Clinical Care." *Academic Medicine* 92 (3). https://doi.org/10.1097/ACM.0000000000001294.

Bourgois, Philippe, and Jeff Schonberg. 2009. *Righteous Dopefiend*. Berkeley: University of California Press.

Braga, Carla Teófilo. 2012. "'Death Is Destiny': Sovereign Decisions and the Lived Experience of HIV/AIDS and Biomedical Treatment in Central Mozambique." PhD diss., State University of New York, Buffalo.

———. 2017. "Producing and Reproducing Inequality: Biopolitical Exclusion, Marginalized Bodies and AIDS Care in Central Mozambique." *Africa Development* 42 (1): 221–43.

Brandt, Allan M. 2013. "How AIDS Invented Global Health." *New England Journal of Medicine* 368 (23): 2149–52. https://doi.org/10.1056/NEJMp1305297.

Brandt, Allan M., and Paul Rozin. 1997. *Morality and Health*. New York: Routledge.

Briggs, Charles L., and Clara Mantini-Briggs. 2003. *Stories in the Time of Cholera: Racial Profiling During a Medical Nightmare*. Berkeley: University of California Press.

Brito, Luís De, Egídio Chaimite, Crescêncio Pereira, Lúcio Posse, Michael Sambo, and Alex Shankland. 2014. *Hunger Revolts and Citizen*

Strikes: Popular Protests in Mozambique, 2008-2012. Brighton, UK: Institute of Development Studies.

Brodish, Paul Henry. 2015. "An Association between Neighbourhood Wealth Inequality and HIV Prevalence in Sub-Saharan Africa." *Journal of Biosocial Science* 47 (3): 311–28. https://doi.org/10.1017 /S0021932013000709.

Brooke, James. 1988. "Maputo Journal: In Marx's Garden; Atheism Wilts, Faith Blooms." *New York Times*, May 10.

Burchardt, Marian. 2015. *Faith in the Time of AIDS: Religion, Biopolitics and Modernity in South Africa*. New York: Palgrave Macmillan.

Burchell, Graham, Colin Gordon, and Peter Miller. 1991. *The Foucault Effect: Studies in Governmentality*. Chicago: University of Chicago Press.

Buur, Lars, and Helene Maria Kyed. 2006. "Contested Sources of Authority: Re-claiming State Sovereignty by Formalizing Traditional Authority in Mozambique." *Development and Change* 37 (4): 847–69.

Cahen, Michel. 2005. "Success in Mozambique?" In *Making States Work: State Failure and the Crisis of Governance*, edited by Simon Chesterman, Michael Ignatieff, Ramesh Chandra Thakur, International Peace Academy, and United Nations University, 213–33. Tokyo: United Nations University Press.

Chapman, Rachel. 2003. "Endangering Safe Motherhood in Mozambique: Prenatal Care as Pregnancy Risk." *Social Science & Medicine* 57: 355–74.

———. 2004. "A Nova Vida: The Commoditization of Reproduction in Central Mozambique." *Medical Anthropology* 23 (3): 229–61.

———. 2006. "Chikotsa—Secrets, Silence, and Hiding: Social Risk and Reproductive Vulnerability in Central Mozambique." *Medical Anthropology Quarterly* 20 (4): 487–515.

———. 2010. *Family Secrets: Risking Reproduction in Central Mozambique*. Nashville, TN: Vanderbilt University Press.

Chavanduka, Gordon. 1978. *Traditional Healers and the Shona Patient*. Gwelo: Mambo Press.

Cliff, Julie. 1991. "The War on Women in Mozambique: Health Consequences of South African Destabilization, Economic Crisis, and Structural Adjustment." In *Woman and Health in Africa*, edited by Meredeth Turshen, 15–33. Trenton, NJ: Africa World Press.

———. 1993. "Donor Dependence or Donor Control? The Case of Mozambique." *Community Development Journal* 28 (3): 237–44.

Cliff, Julie, and A. R. Noormahomed. 1988. "Health as a Target: South Africa's Destabilization of Mozambique." *Social Science & Medicine* 27 (7): 717–22.

Collins, Carole. 2006. *Mozambique's HIV/AIDS Pandemic: Grappling with Apartheid's Legacy.* Edited by UNRISD, Social Policy and Development Programme. Geneva: United National Research Institute for Social Development.

Comaroff, Jean. 1982. "Medicine: Symbol and Ideology." In *The Problem of Medical Knowledge: Examining the Social Construction of Medicine,* edited by Peter Wright and Andrew Treacher, 49–69. Edinburgh: Edinburgh University Press.

———. 1985. *Body of Power, Spirit of Resistance: The Culture and History of a South African People.* Chicago: University of Chicago Press.

Comaroff, Jean, and John Comaroff. 2012. "Theory from the South: Or, How Euro-America Is Evolving toward Africa." *Anthropological Forum* 22 (2): 113–31. https://doi.org/10.1080/00664677.2012.694169.

Comaroff, Jean, and John L. Comaroff. 1999. "Occult Economies and the Violence of Abstraction: Notes from the South African Postcolony." *American Ethnologist* 26 (2): 279–303. https://doi.org/10.1525/ae.1999.26.2.279.

Comaroff, John L., and Jean Comaroff. 1999. "On Personhood: An Anthropological Perspective from Africa." ABF Working Paper, no. 9903, Chicago, American Bar Foundation.

Conselho Nacional De Combate Ao HIV/SIDA [National Council for the Fight Against HIV/AIDS]. 2004. *Plano estratégico nacional de combate ao HIV/SIDA* [National strategic plan for the fight against HIV/AIDS. Maputo: Conselho Nacional De Combate Ao HIV/SIDA.

Costello, Daniel. 2008. "HIV Treatment Becoming Profitable." *Los Angeles Times,* February 21. www.latimes.com/business/la-fi-hiv21feb21,1,6460362.story.

Craddock, Susan. 2004. "Beyond Epidemiology: Locating AIDS in Africa." In *HIV and AIDS in Africa: Beyond Epidemiology,* edited by Ezekiel Kalipeni, Susan Craddock, Joseph R. Oppong, and Jayati Ghosh, 1–14. Malden, MA: Blackwell.

Cramer, Christopher. 2001. "Privatisation and Adjustment in Mozambique: A 'Hospital Pass?'" *Journal of Southern African Studies* 27 (1): 79–103. https://doi.org/10.1080/03057070120029518.

———. 2007. *Violence in Developing Countries: War, Memory, Progress.* Bloomington: Indiana University Press.

Crane, Johanna Tayloe. 2013. *Scrambling for Africa: AIDS, Expertise, and the Rise of American Global Health Science*. Ithaca, NY: Cornell University Press.

Crimp, Douglas. 1988. "AIDS: Cultural Analysis/Cultural Activism." In *AIDS: Cultural Analysis/Cultural Activism*, 3–16. Cambridge, MA: MIT Press.

Cruikshank, Barbara. 1993. "Revolutions Within: Self-Government and Self-Esteem." *Economy and Society* 22 (3): 327–44.

Cruz e Silva, Teresa. 2001a. "Entre a exclusão social e o exercício da cidadania: Igrejas 'Zione' do bairro Luís Cabral, na cidade de Maputo." *Estudos Moçambicanos*, no. 19: 27–60.

Cruz e Silva, Teresa. 2001b. *Protestant Churches and the Formation of Political Consciousness in Southern Mozambique (1930–1974)*. Basel, Switzerland: P. Schlettwein.

Cunguara, Benedito, and Joseph Hanlon. 2010. "Poverty Is Not Being Reduced in Mozambique." Crisis States Research Centre Working Papers Series no. 2, Working Paper no. 74. www.lse.ac.uk/international -development/Assets/Documents/PDFs/csrc-working-papers-phase -two/wp74.2-poverty-is-not-being-reduced-mozambique.pdf.

D'Adesky, Anne-Christine. 2006. *Moving Mountains: The Race to Treat Global AIDS*. New York: Verso Books.

Davis, Mike. 2004. "Planet of Slums." *New Left Review* 26 (March–April): 5–34.

Dijk, Rijk Van, Hansjorg Dilger, Marian Burchardt, and Theresa Rasing. 2014. *Religion and AIDS Treatment in Africa: Saving Souls, Prolonging Lives*. Burlington: Ashgate.

Dilger, Hansjörg. 2001. "'Living PositHIVely in Tanzania'. The Global Dynamics of AIDS and the Meaning of Religion for International and Local AIDS Work." *Afrika Spectrum* 1: 73–90.

———. 2007. "Healing the Wounds of Modernity: Salvation, Community and Care in a Neo-Pentecostal Church in Dar Es Salaam, Tanzania." *Journal of Religion in Africa*, no. 37: 59–83.

———. 2010. "'My Relatives Are Running Away from Me!' Kinship and Care in the Wake of Structural Adjustment, Privatization, and HIV/AIDS in Tanzania." In *Anthropologies of AIDS: The Morality of Illness, Treatment, and Death in Africa*, edited by Hansjörg Dilger and Ute Luig, 102–24. New York: Berghahn Books.

———. 2012. "Targeting the Empowered Individual: Transnational Policy Making, the Global Economy of Aid, and the Limitations of Biopower in Tanzania." In *Medicine, Mobility, and Power in Global Africa*, edited by Hansjörg Dilger, Abdoulaye Kane, and Stacey A. Langwick, 60–91. Bloomington: Indiana University Press.

Drewes, S. E., and F. Khan. 2004. "The African Potato (Hypoxis Hemerocallidea): A Chemical–Historical Perspective." *South Africa Journal of Science* (October): 425–30.

Droggitis, Christina, and Nandini Oomman. 2010. "Think Long Term: How Global AIDS Donors Can Strengthen the Health Workforce in Africa." Center for Global Development. www.cgdev.org/publication /think-long-term-how-global-aids-donors-can-strengthen-health -workforce-africa.

Dubal, Sam. 2012. "Renouncing Paul Farmer: A Desperate Plea for Radical Political Medicine." *Being Ethical in an Unethical World* (blog). May 27. http://samdubal.blogspot.com/2012/05/renouncing-paul-farmer -desperate-plea.html.

———. 2018. *Against Humanity: Lessons from the Lord's Resistance Army*. Oakland: University of California Press.

Dube, Francis. 2009. "Colonialism, Cross-Border Movements , and Epidemiology: A History of Public Health in the Manica Region of Central Mozambique and Eastern Zimbabwe and the African Response, 1890-1980." PhD diss., University of Iowa.

———. 2015. "'In the Border Regions of the Territory of Rhodesia, There Is the Greatest Scourge . . .': The Border and East Coast Fever Control in Central Mozambique and Eastern Zimbabwe, 1901–1942.'" *Journal of Southern African Studies* 41 (2): 219–35. https://doi.org/10.1080 /03057070.2015.1012904.

Dumont, Louis. 1977. *From Mandeville to Marx: The Genesis and Triumph of Economic Ideology*. Chicago: University of Chicago Press.

Durevall, Dick, and Annika Lindskog. 2012. "Economic Inequality and HIV in Malawi." *World Development* 40 (7): 1435–51. https://doi.org /10.1016/j.worlddev.2011.12.003.

Edelman, Marc. 2012. "E. P. Thompson and Moral Economies." In *A Companion to Moral Anthropology*, edited by Didier Fassin, 49–66. Malden, MA: Wiley-Blackwell. https://doi.org/10.1002/9781118290 620.ch3.

Elisha, Omri. 2008. "Moral Ambitions of Grace: The Paradox of Compassion and Accountability in Evangelical Faith-Based Activism." *Cultural Anthropology* 23 (1): 154–89. https://doi.org/10.1111/j.1548-1360.2008 .00006.x.

England, Roger. 2007. "The Dangers of Disease Specific Aid Programmes."
   British Medical Journal 335 (September 15): 565.
Englund, Harri. 1996. "Witchcraft, Modernity and the Person: The
   Morality of Accumulation in Central Malawi." *Critique of Anthro-
   pology* 16 (3): 257–79. https://doi.org/10.1177/0308275X9601600303.
———. 2006. *Prisoners of Freedom.* Berkeley: University of California
   Press.
Epstein, Helen. 2007. *The Invisible Cure: Africa, the West, and the Fight
   Against AIDS.* 1st ed. New York: Farrar, Straus and Giroux.
Epstein, Steven. 1996. *Impure Science: AIDS, Activism, and the Politics of
   Knowledge.* Medicine and Society. Berkeley: University of California
   Press. http://ark.cdlib.org/ark:/13030/ft1s20045x/.
Fanon, Frantz. 1961. *The Wretched of the Earth.* New York: Grove Press.
———. 1965. *A Dying Colonialism.* New York: Grove Press.
———. 1967. *Black Skin, White Masks.* New York: Grove Press.
Farmer, Paul. 1988. "Bad Blood, Spoiled Milk: Bodily Fluids as Moral
   Barometers in Rural Haiti." *American Ethnologist* 15 (1): 62–83.
———. 1992. *AIDS and Accusation: Haiti and the Geography of Blame.*
   Berkeley: University of California Press.
———. 1999. *Infections and Inequalities: The Modern Plagues.* Berkeley:
   University of California Press.
———. 2004. "An Anthropology of Structural Violence." *Current Anthro-
   pology* 45 (3): 305–25.
Farmer, Paul, F. Leandre, J. S. Mukherjee, M. S. Claude, P. Nevil, and
   M. C. Smith-Fawzi. 2001. "Community-Based Approaches to HIV
   Treatment in Resource-Poor Settings." *Lancet*, no. 358: 404–9.
Farmer, Paul, Jim Yong Kim, Arthur Kleinman, and Matthew Basilico.
   2013. *Reimagining Global Health: An Introduction.* Berkeley: University of California Press.
Fassin, Didier. 2001. "Culturalism as Ideology." In *Cultural Perspectives
   on Reproductive Health*, edited by Carla Makhlouf Obermeyer,
   300–317. Oxford: Oxford University Press.
———. 2007. *When Bodies Remember: Experiences and Politics of AIDS
   in South Africa.* Berkeley: University of California Press.
———. 2009. "Moral Economies Revisited." *Annales. Histoire, Sciences
   Sociales* 64 (6): 1237–66.
———. 2012. *Humanitarian Reason: A Moral History of the Present.*
   Berkeley: University of California Press.

Feierman, Steven. 1985. "Struggles for Control: The Social Roots of Health and Healing in Modern Africa." *African Studies Review* 28 (2–3): 73–147.

———. 2006. "Afterword: Ethnographic Regions—Healing, Power, and History." In *Borders and Healers: Brokering Therapeutic Resources in Southeast Africa*, edited by Tracy Luedke and Harry G West, 185–94. Bloomington: Indiana University Press.

Feierman, Steven, and John M Janzen. 1992. *The Social Basis of Health and Healing in Africa*. Berkeley: University of California Press.

Feinglass, Ellie, Nadja Gomes, and Vivek Maru. 2016. "Transforming Policy into Justice: The Role of Health Advocates in Mozambique." *Health and Human Rights* 18 (2): 233–46.

Ferguson, James. 1990. *The Anti-Politics Machine: "Development," Depoliticization, and Bureaucratic Power in Lesotho*. New York: Cambridge University Press.

———. 2006. *Global Shadows: Africa in the Neoliberal World Order*. Durham, NC: Duke University Press.

———. 2013. "Declarations of Dependence: Labour, Personhood, and Welfare in Southern Africa." *Journal of the Royal Anthropological Institute* 19: 223–42. https://doi.org/10.1111/1467-9655.12023.

———. 2015. *Give a Man a Fish: Reflections on the New Politics of Distribution*. Durham, NC: Duke University Press.

Ferguson, James, and Akhil Gupta. 2002. "Spatializing States: Toward an Ethnography of Neoliberal Governmentality." *American Ethnologist*, no. 2: 981–1002.

Finnegan, William. 1993. *A Complicated War: The Harrowing of Mozambique*. Perspectives on Southern Africa. Berkeley: University of California Press.

Fontaine, J. S. La. 1985. "Person and Individual: Some Anthropological Reflections." In *The Category of the Person: Anthropology, Philosophy, History*, edited by Michael Carrithers, Steven Collins, and Steven Lukes, 123–40. Cambridge, UK: Cambridge University Press.

Fort, Meredith, Mary Anne Mercer, Oscar Gish, and Steven Gloyd. 2004. *Sickness and Wealth: The Corporate Assault on Global Health*. Cambridge: South End Press.

Fortes, Meyer. 1987. "The Concept of the Person." In *Religion, Morality, and the Person: Essays on Tallensi Religion*, 247–86. New York: Cambridge University Press.

Foster, George M. 1976. "Disease Etiologies in Non-Western Medical Systems." *American Anthropologist* 78 (4): 773–82.

Foucault, Michel. 1990. *The History of Sexuality*. New York: Vintage Books.

———. 1991. "Governmentality." In *The Foucault Effect: Studies in Governmentality*, edited by Graham Burchell, Colin Gordon, and Peter Miller, 87–104. Chicago: University of Chicago Press.

———. 2003. *"Society Must Be Defended": Lectures at the Collège de France, 1975–76*. Edited by Arnold I Davidson. 1st ed. New York: Picador.

———. 2008. *The Birth of Biopolitics: Lectures at the College de France, 1978–79*. Edited by Michel Senellart. New York: Palgrave Macmillan.

FRELIMO. 1979. *Xiconhoca—O Inimigo*. Maputo: Departamento do Trabalho Ideológico da FRELIMO.

Fry, Peter. 2000. "O espírito santo contra o feitiço e os espíritos revoltados: 'Civilização' e 'tradição' em Moçambique." *Mana* 6 (2): 65–95.

Garrido, Juan Manuel. 2012. *On Time, Being, and Hunger*. New York City: Fordham University Press.

Geffray, C. 1990. *La cause des armes au Mozambique: Anthropologie d'un guerre civile*. Nairobi: Credu-Karthala.

Gerety, Rowan Moore. 2018. *Go Tell the Crocodiles: Chasing Prosperity in Mozambique*. New York: New Press.

Gershon, Ilana. 2011. "Neoliberal Agency." *Current Anthropology* 52 (4): 537–55. https://doi.org/10.1086/660866.

Geschiere, Peter. 1997. *The Modernity of Witchcraft: Politics and the Occult in Postcolonial Africa*. Charlottesville: University Press of Virginia.

Gillespie, Stuart. 2006. *AIDS, Poverty, and Hunger: Challenges and Responses*. Washington, DC: International Food Policy Research Institute.

Gimbel, Sarah, Baltazar Chilundo, Nora Kenworthy, Celso Inguane, David Citrin, Rachel Chapman, Kenneth Sherr, and James Pfeiffer. 2018. "Donor Data Vacuuming: Audit Culture and the Use of Data in Global Heath Partnerships." *Medicine Anthropology Theory* 5 (2): 99. https://doi.org/10.17157/mat.5.2.537.

Giridharadas, Anand. 2018. *Winners Take All: The Elite Charade of Changing the World*. New York: Alfred A. Knopf.

Glasgow, Sara, and Ted Schrecker. 2016. "The Double Burden of Neoliberalism? Noncommunicable Disease Policies and the Global Political

Economy of Risk." *Health and Place* 39 (May): 204–11. https://doi.org/10.1016/j.healthplace.2016.04.003.

Gloyd, Stephen, James Pfeiffer, and Wendy Johnson. 2013. "Cooperantes, Solidarity, and the Fight for Health in Mozambique." In *Comrades in Health: U.S. Health Internationalists, Abroad and at Home*, 184–99. New Brunswick, NJ: Rutgers University Press.

Gloyd, Steven. 1996. "NGOs and the "SAP"Ing of Health Care in Rural Mozambique." *Hesperian Foundation News* (Spring).

Gluckman, Max. 1956. *Custom and Conflict in Africa*. Oxford: Blackwell.

Gray, Dylan Mohan. 2013. *Fire in the Blood*. Mumbai: International Film Circuit.

Grebe, Eduard. 2011. "The Treatment Action Campaign's Struggle for Aids Treatment in South Africa: Coalition-Building through Networks." *Journal of Southern African Studies* 37 (4): 849–68. https://doi.org/10.1080/03057070.2011.608271.

Green, E. C. 1996. "Purity, Pollution and the Invisible Snake in Southern Africa." *Medical Anthropology* 17 (1): 83–100. https://doi.org/10.1080/01459740.1996.9966129.

Greene, Jeremy, Marguerite Thorp Basilico, Heidi Kim, and Paul Farmer. 2013. "Colonial Medicine and Its Legacies." In *Reimagining Global Health: An Introduction*, edited by Paul Farmer, Jim Yong Kim, Arthur Kleinman, and Matthew Basilico, 33–73. Berkeley: University of California Press.

Guerreiro, Manuela Sousa. 2003. "Textáfrica está à venda." *Moçambique* 34: 37–38.

Gusdal, Annelie K., Celestino Obua, Tenaw Andualem, Rolf Wahlström, Göran Tomson, Stefan Peterson, Anna Mia Ekström, Anna Thorson, John Chalker, and Grethe Fochsen. 2009. "Voices on Adherence to ART in Ethiopia and Uganda: A Matter of Choice or Simply Not an Option?" *AIDS Care—Psychological and Socio-Medical Aspects of AIDS/HIV* 21 (11): 1381–87. https://doi.org/10.1080/09540120902883119.

Guyer, Jane I. 1993. "Wealth in People and Self-Realization in Equatorial Africa." *Man* 28 (2): 243–65. https://doi.org/10.2307/2803412.

Hacking, Ian. 1986. "Making Up People." In *Reconstructing Individualism: Autonomy, Individuality, and the Self in Western Thought*, edited by Thomas C. Heller, Morton Sosna, Christine Brooke-Rose, and David E. Wellbery, 222–36. Palo Alto, CA: Stanford University Press.

Hanlon, Joseph. 1990. *Mozambique: The Revolution under Fire*. London: Zed Books.

———. 1991. *Mozambique: Who Calls the Shots?* Bloomington: Indiana University Press.

———. 1996. *Peace without Profit: How the IMF Blocks Rebuilding in Mozambique.* Portsmouth, NH: Heinemann.

———. 1999. "Two Decades of Competition over Health in Mozambique." In *Managing Development: Understanding Inter-organizational Relationships*, edited by Dorcas Robinson, Tom Hewitt, and John Harris, 115–35. n.p.: Sage Publications.

———. 2007. "Is Poverty Decreasing in Mozambique?" In *Inaugural Conference of the Instituto de Estudos Sociais e Económicos*, 15. Maputo: Instituto de Estudos Sociais e Económicos.

———. 2009. "Just Give Money to the Poor." In *Dinamicas da pobreza e padrões de acumulação em Moçambique*,10. Maputo: Instituto de Estudos Sociais e Económicos.

———. 2020a. "Notes on the Evolution of the Cabo Delgado War: Although the Global Should Not Be Forgotten, the Local Is Most Important." *Mozambique News Reports & Clippings*, February 27.

———. 2020b. "$ 5.7 Bn Loans to Support 18, 700 Jobs in US, UK." *Mozambique News Reports & Clippings*, July 2.

Hanlon, Joseph, Armando Barrientos, and David Hulme. 2010. *Just Give Money to the Poor: The Development Revolution from the Global South.* Sterling, VA: Kumarian Press.

Hanlon, Joseph, and Teresa Smart. 2008. *Do Bicycles Equal Development in Mozambique?* Rochester, NY: James Currey.

Hardiman, David. 2006. *Healing Bodies, Saving Souls. Medical Missions in Asia and Africa.* Amsterdam: Editions Rodopi B.V.

Harries, A. D., D. S. Nyangulu, N. J. Hargreaves, O. Kaluwa, and F. M. Salaniponi. 2001. "Preventing Antiretroviral Anarchy in Sub-Saharan Africa." *Lancet* 358: 410–14. https://doi.org/10.1016/S0140-6736(01)05551-9.

Harrington, Anne. 2008. *The Cure Within: A History of Mind-Body Medicine.* New York: W. W. Norton.

Hearing on the United States' War on AIDS before the House Committee on International Relations. 2001. 107th Cong., 1st Sess. (June 7) (testimony of Andrew Natsios). http://commdocs.house.gov/committees/intlrel/hfa72978.000/hfa72978_0.HTM.

Helgesson, A. 1994. *Church, State, and People in Mozambique.* Uppsala: Uppsala University, Swedish Institute of Missionary Research.

Høg, Erling. 2008. "The Process: Experiences, Limitations, and Politics of ARV Treatment in Mozambique." PhD diss., London School of Economics and Political Science.

———. 2014. "HIV Scale-up in Mozambique: Exceptionalism, Normalisation and Global Health." *Global Public Health* 9 (1–2): 210–23. https://doi.org/10.1080/17441692.2014.881522.

Holland, Dorothy, and Kevin Leander. 2004. "Ethnographic Studies of Positioning and Subjectivity: An Introduction." *Ethos* 32 (2): 127–39. https://doi.org/10.1525/eth.2004.32.2.127.

Holmes, Seth M., Jeremy A. Greene, and Scott D. Stonington. 2014. "Locating Global Health in Social Medicine." *Global Public Health* 9 (5): 475–80. https://doi.org/10.1080/17441692.2014.897361.

Honwana, Alcinda. 1996. "Spiritual Agency & Self-Renewal in Southern Mozambique," PhD diss., School of Oriental and African Studies University of London.

———. 2002. *Espíritos vivos, tradições modernas: Possessão de espíritos e reintegração social pos-guerra no sul de Moçambique.* Colecção identidades. Maputo: Promédia.

Horton, Richard. 2018. "Offline: Frantz Fanon and the Origins of Global Health." *Lancet* 392 (10149): 720. https://doi.org/10.1016/S0140-6736(18)32041-5.

Huhn, Arianna. 2016. "What Is Human? Anthropomorphic Anthropophagy in Northwest Mozambique." In *Cooking Cultures: Convergent Histories of Food and Feeling*, 177–98. Cambridge, UK: Cambridge University Press.

Hunter, Mark. 2010. *Love in the Time of AIDS: Inequality, Gender and Right in South Africa.* Bloomington: Indiana University Press.

Iliffe, John. 2006. *The African AIDS Epidemic: A History.* Oxford: James Currey.

International Labour Organization. 2012. *R202-Social Protection Floors Recommendation, 2012 (No. 202).* www.ilo.org/dyn/normlex/en/f?p=NORMLEXPUB:12100:0::NO::P12100_INSTRUMENT_ID:3065524.

International Monetary Fund (IMF). 2016. "Republic of Mozambique—Selected Issues." *IMF Country Report*(January): 1–29. www.imf.org/external/pubs/ft/scr/2016/cr10.pdf.

Isaacman, Allen. 1975. "The Tradition of Resistance in Mozambique." *Africa Today* 22 (3): 37–50.

———. 1996. *Cotton Is the Mother of Poverty: Peasants, Work, and Rural Struggle in Colonial Mozambique, 1938–1961*. Social History of Africa. Portsmouth, NH: Heinemann.

Isaacman, Allen, and Barbara Isaacman. 1976. *The Tradition of Resistance in Mozambique: Anti-Colonial Activity in the Zambesi Valley, 1850–1921*. London: Heinemann.

———. 1983. *Mozambique: From Colonialism to Revolution, 1900–1982*. Boulder, CO: Westview Press.

Isaacman, Allen, and Chris Sneddon. 2000. "Toward a Social and Environmental History of the Building of Cahora Bassa Dam." *Journal of Southern African Studies* 26 (4): 597–632.

Janzen, John M. 1978. *The Quest for Therapy in Lower Zaire*. Berkeley: University of California Press.

Jobarteh, Kebba, Ray W. Shiraishi, Inacio Malimane, Paula Samo Gudo, Tom Decroo, Andrew F. Auld, Vania Macome, and Aleny Couto. 2016. "Community ART Support Groups in Mozambique: The Potential of Patients as Partners in Care." *PLoS ONE* 11 (12): 1–14. https://doi.org /10.1371/journal.pone.0166444.

Kadiyala, Suneetha, Rahul Rawat, Terry Roopnaraine, Frances Babirye, and Robert Ochai. 2009. "Applying a Programme Theory Framework to Improve Livelihood Interventions Integrated with HIV Care and Treatment Programmes." *Journal of Development Effectiveness* 1 (4): 470–91. https://doi.org/10.1080/19439340903370469.

Kalofonos, Ippolytos. 2008. "'All I Eat Is ARVs': Living with HIV/AIDS at the Dawn of the Treatment Era in Central Mozambique." PhD diss., University of California, San Francisco.

———. 2010. "'All I Eat Is ARVs': The Paradox of AIDS Treatment Interventions in Central Mozambique." *Medical Anthropology Quarterly* 24 (3): 363–80. https://doi.org/10.1111/j.1548-1387.2010.01109.x.

———. 2019. "Biological Citizenship—A 53-Year-Old Man with Schizo-affective Disorder and PTSD Applying for Supplemental Security Income." *New England Journal of Medicine* 381 (21): 1985–89.

Karandinos, George, Laurie Kain Hart, Fernando Montero Castrillo, and Philippe Bourgois. 2014. "The Moral Economy of Violence in the US Inner City." *Current Anthropology* 55 (1): 1–22. https://doi.org/10.1086 /674613.

Karp, Ivan. 1997. "Notions of Person." In *Encyclopedia of Africa South of the Sahara*, edited by John Middleton, 392–96. New York: C. Scribner's Sons.

Keller, Richard C. 2006. "Geographies of Power, Legacies of Mistrust: Colonial Medicine in the Global Present." *Historical Geography* 34: 26–48.

Kelley, Maureen, Rashida Ferrand, Kui Muraya, Simukai Chigudu, Sassy Molyneux, Madhukar Pai, and Edwine Barasa. 2020. "An Appeal to Practical Social Justice in the COVID-19 Global Response in Low-Income and Middle-Income Countries." *Lancet: Global Health* 8 (7): e888–89. https://doi.org/10.1016/S2214-109X(20)30249-7.

Kentikelenis, Alexander E., Thomas H. Stubbs, and Lawrence P. King. 2015. "Structural Adjustment and Public Spending on Health: Evidence from IMF Programs in Low-Income Countries." *Social Science and Medicine* 126: 169–76. https://doi.org/10.1016/j.socscimed.2014.12.027.

Kenworthy, Nora J., and Richard Parker. 2014. "HIV Scale-up and the Politics of Global Health: Introduction." *Global Public Health* 9 (1–2): 1–6. https://doi.org/10.1080/17441692.2014.880727.

Kenworthy, Nora J., Matthew Thomann, and Richard Parker. 2017. "From a Global Crisis to the 'End of AIDS': New Epidemics of Signification." *Global Public Health* 13 (8): 960–71. https://doi.org/10.1080/17441692.2017.1365373.

Keshavjee, Salmaan. 2014. *Blind Spot: How Neoliberalism Infiltrated Global Health.* Oakland: University of California Press.

Kim, Jim Yong, Joyce V. Millen, Alec Irwin, and John Gershman. 2000. *Dying for Growth: Global Inequality and the Health of the Poor.* Series in Health and Social Justice. Monroe, ME: Common Courage Press.

King, Nicholas B. 2002. "Ideologies of Postcolonial Global Health." *Social Studies of Science* 32 (5–6) (October–December): 763–89.

Klaits, Frederick. 2010. *Death in a Church of Life: Moral Passion during Botswana's Time of AIDS.* Berkeley: University of California Press.

Kleinman, Arthur. 1995. *Writing at the Margin: Discourse between Anthropology and Medicine.* Berkeley: University of California Press.

———. 2012. "Caregiving as Moral Experience." *Lancet* 380 (9853): 1550–51. https://doi.org/10.1016/S0140-6736(12)61870-4.

———. 2015. "Care: In Search of a Health Agenda." *Lancet* 386 (9990): 240–41. https://doi.org/10.1016/S0140-6736(15)61271-5.

Kleinman, Arthur, and Bridget Hanna. 2008. "Catastrophe, Caregiving and Today's Biomedicine." *BioSocieties* 3 (3): 287–301. https://doi.org/10.1017/S1745855208006200.

Koenig, S. P., F. Leandre, and P. E. Farmer. 2004. "Scaling-up HIV Treatment Programmes in Resource-Limited Settings: The Rural Haiti Experience." *AIDS* 18 (Supp. 3): S21–5.

Kothari, Uma. 2006. "An Agenda for Thinking about 'Race' in Development." *Progress in Development Studies* 6 (1): 9–23. https://doi.org/10.1191/1464993406ps124oa.

Kuehn, Kathleen, and Thomas F. Corrigan. 2013. "Hope Labor: The Role of Employment Prospects in Online Social Production." *Political Economy of Communication* 1 (1): 9–25.

Kyed, Helene Maria. 2007. "The Politics of Policing: Re-Capturing 'Zones of Confusion' in Rural Post-War Mozambique." In *The Security-Development Nexus: Expressions of Sovereignty and Securitization in Southern Africa*, edited by Lars Buur, Steffen Jensen, and Finn Stepputat, 132–51. Cape Town: HSRC Press.

Lambdin, Barrot H., Mark A. Micek, Kenneth Sherr, Sarah Gimbel, Marina Karagianis, Joseph Lara, Stephen S. Gloyd, and James Pfeiffer. 2013. "Integration of HIV Care and Treatment in Primary Health Care Centers and Patient Retention in Central Mozambique: A Retrospective Cohort Study." *Journal of Acquired Immune Deficiency Syndromes* 62 (5): 146–52. https://doi.org/10.1097/QAI.0b013e3182840d4e.

Lan, David. 1985. *Guns & Rain: Guerrillas & Spirit Mediums in Zimbabwe*. Berkeley: University of California Press.

Lancet Editorial. 2020. "Food Insecurity Will Be the Sting in the Tail of COVID-19." *Lancet: Global Health* 8 (6): e737. https://doi.org/10.1016/S2214-109X(20)30228-X.

Langwick, Stacey A. 2011. *Bodies, Politics, and African Healing : The Matter of Maladies in Tanzania*. Bloomington: Indiana University Press.

Lehmann, Uta, and David Sanders. 2007. *Community Health Workers: What Do We Know about Them?* Geneva: World Health Organization.

Livingston, Julie. 2005. *Debility and the Moral Imagination in Botswana*. African Systems of Thought. Bloomington: Indiana University Press.

———. 2012. *Improvising Medicine: An African Oncology Ward in an Emerging Cancer Epidemic*. Durham, NC: Duke University Press.

Lock, Margaret M., and Vinh-Kim Nguyen. 2010. *An Anthropology of Biomedicine*. Malden, MA: Wiley-Blackwell.

Lubega, Muhamadi, Xavier Nsabagasani, Nazarius M. Tumwesigye, Fred Wabwire-Mangen, Anna Mia Ekström, George Pariyo, and Stefan

Peterson. 2010. "Policy and Practice, Lost in Transition: Reasons for High Drop-out from Pre-antiretroviral Care in a Resource-Poor Setting of Eastern Uganda." *Health Policy* 95: 153–58. https://doi.org/10.1016/j.healthpol.2009.11.021.

Lubkemann, Stephen C. 2001. "Rebuilding Local Capacities in Mozambique: The National Health System and Civil Society." In *Patronage or Partnership: Local Capacity Building in Humanitarian Crises*, edited by Ian Smillie, 77–106. Bloomfield, CT: Kumarian Press.

Luedke, Tracy. 2007. "Spirit and Matter: The Materiality of Mozambican Prophet Healing." *Journal of Southern African Studies* 33 (4): 715–31. https://doi.org/10.1080/03057070701646779.

Luhrmann, Tanya. 2006. "Subjectivity." *Anthropological Theory* 6 (3): 345–61.

Macamo, Elísio. 2005. "How Development Aid Changes Societies: Disciplining Mozambique Through Structural Adjustment." In *11th CODESRIA General Assembly, Rethinking African Development: Beyond Impasse, towards Alternatives*. Maputo: CODESRIA. http://codesria.org/Links/conferences/general_assembly11/papers/macamo.pdf.

———. 2006. "HIV." *Meianoite*, July 26, 2.

———. 2017. "Power, Conflict, and Citizenship: Mozambique's Contemporary Struggles." *Citizenship Studies* 21 (2): 196–209. https://doi.org/10.1080/13621025.2017.1279796.

Machel, Samora. 1976. "Hospital Speech." Special issue, *Boletim—A Saude en Mozambique* (October).

———. 1985. *Samora Machel, an African Revolutionary: Selected Speeches and Writings*. Edited by Barry Munslow. London: Zed Books.

Maes, Kenneth. 2012. "Volunteerism or Labor Exploitation ? Harnessing the Volunteer Spirit to Sustain AIDS Treatment Programs in Urban Ethiopia." *Human Organization* 71 (1): 54.

———. 2016. *The Lives of Community Health Workers: Local Labor and Global Health in Urban Ethiopia*. New York: Routledge. https://doi.org/10.4324/9781315400785.

Maes, Kenneth, Svea Closser, and Ippolytos Kalofonos. 2014. "Listening to Community Health Workers: How Ethnographic Research Can Inform Positive Relationships among Community Health Workers, Health Institutions, and Communities." *American Journal of Public Health* 104 (5): e5–9. https://doi.org/10.2105/AJPH.2014.301907.

Maes, Kenneth, and Ippolytos Kalofonos. 2013. "Becoming and Remaining Community Health Workers: Perspectives from Ethiopia and

Mozambique." *Social Science & Medicine* 87: 52–59. https://doi.org/10
.1016/j.socscimed.2013.03.026.

Maes, Kenneth, and Selamawit Shifferaw. 2011. "Cycles of Poverty, Food
Insecurity, and Psychosocial Stress among AIDS Care Volunteers in
Urban Ethiopia." In "HIV/AIDS and Food Insecurity in Sub-Saharan
Africa: Challenges and Solutions." Special issue, *Annals of Anthropo-
logical Practice* 35: 98–115. https://doi.org/http://dx.doi.org/10.1111/j
.2153-9588.2011.01069.x.

Maeseneer, Jan De, Chris van Weel, David Egilman, Khaya Mfenyana,
Arthur Kaufman, and Nelson Sewankambo. 2008. "Strengthening
Primary Care: Addressing the Disparity between Vertical and Horizontal Investment." *British Journal of General Practice* 58 (546): 3–4.
https://doi.org/10.3399/bjgp08X263721.

Mahoney, Michael. 2003. "Estado Novo, Homem Novo (New State, New
Man): Colonial and Anticolonial Development Ideologies in Mozambique, 1930–1977." In *Staging Growth: Modernization, Development,
and the Global Cold War*, 165–97. Amherst: University of Massachu-
setts Press.

Mamdani, Mahmood. 1996. *Citizen and Subject: Contemporary Africa
and the Legacy of Late Colonialism*. Princeton, NJ: Princeton University Press.

Manning, Carrie. 1998. "Constructing Opposition in Mozambique:
Renamo as Political Party." *Journal of Southern African Studies* 24 (1):
161–89.

Marks, Shula. 2002. "An Epidemic Waiting to Happen? The Spread of
HIV/AIDS in South Africa in Social and Historical Perspective."
Journal of Southern African Studies 61 (1): 13–26.

Markus, Hazel Rose, and Shinobu Kitayama. 1991. "Culture and the Self:
Implications for Cognition, Emotion, and Motivation." *Psychological
Review* 98 (2): 224–53. https://doi.org/10.1037/0033-295X.98.2.224.

Marsland, Rebecca. 2012. "(Bio)Sociality and HIV in Tanzania: Finding a
Living to Support a Life." *Medical Anthropology Quarterly* 26: 470–85.
https://doi.org/10.1111/maq.12002.

Matsinhe, Cristiano. 2005. *Tábula rasa: Dinâmica da resposta Moçambicana ao HIV/SIDA*. Maputo: Texto Editores.

Mavie, Gustavo. 2007. "Falta de hábito ao trabalho perpetua fome no
país—considera Presidente Armando Guebuza" [Lack of work ethic
perpetuates hunger in the country–according to President Armando
Guebuza]. *Notícias*, April 19.

Maxwell, David. 2002. "Christianity without Frontiers: Shona Missionaries and Transnational Pentecostalism in Africa." In *Christianity and the African Imagination: Essays in Honour of Adrian Hastings*, edited by Adrian Hastings, David Maxwell, and Ingrid Lawrie, 295–332. Leiden: Brill.

Mbembe, Achille. 2001. *On the Postcolony*. Studies on the History of Society and Culture, no. 41. Berkeley: University of California Press.

———. 2017. *Critique of Black Reason*. Durham, NC: Duke University Press.

———. 2019. *Necropolitics*. Durham, NC: Duke University Press.

McKay, Ramah. 2012. "Documentary Disorders: Managing Medical Multiplicity in Maputo, Mozambique." *American Ethnologist* 39 (3): 545–61. https://doi.org/10.1111/j.1548-1425.2012.01380.x.

McKay, Ramah. 2018. *Medicine in the Meantime: The Work of Care in Mozambique*. Durham, NC: Duke University Press.

Meneses, Maria Paula. 2007. "'When There Are No Problems, We Are Healthy, No Bad Luck, Nothing': Towards an Emancipatory Understanding of Health and Medicine." In *Another Knowledge Is Possible: Beyond Northern Epistemologies*, edited by Boaventura de Sousa Santos, 352–80. New York: Verso.

Meneses, Maria Paula. 2015. "Xiconhoca, o inimigo: Narrativas de violência sobre a construção da nação em Moçambique" [Xiconhoca, the enemy: Narratives of violence about the construction of the nation in Mozambique]. *Revista Crítica de Ciências Sociais*, no. 106: 9–52. https://doi.org/10.4000/rccs.5869.

Messac, Luke, and Krishna Prabhu. 2013. "Redefining the Possible: The Global AIDS Response." In *Reimagining Global Health: An Introduction*, edited by Paul Farmer, Jim Yong Kim, Arthur Kleinman, and Matthew Basilico, 111–32. Oakland: University of California Press.

Metzl, Jonathan M, and Helena Hansen. 2014. "Structural Competency: Theorizing a New Medical Engagement with Stigma and Inequality." *Social Science & Medicine* 103: 126–33. https://doi.org/10.1016/j.socscimed.2013.06.032.

Meyer, Birgit. 1998. "'Make a Complete Break with the Past': Memory and Post-Colonial Modernity in Ghanaian Pentecostalist Discourse'." *Journal of Religion in Africa* 28: 316–49. https://doi.org/10.1163/157006698X00044.

———. 2004. "Christianity in Africa: From African Independent to Pentecostal-Charismatic Churches." *Annual Review of Anthropology* 33: 447–74. https://doi.org/10.1146/annurev.anthro.33.070203.143835.

Miers, Suzanne, and Igor Kopytoff. 1977. *Slavery in Africa: Historical and Anthropological Perspectives*. Madison: University of Wisconsin Press.

MISAU. 2005. *Relatório sobre a revisão dos dados de vigilância epidemiológica do HIV—ronda 2004*. Maputo: República De Moçambique, Ministério de Saúde, Direcção Nacional de Saúde.

———. 2006. *Manual do formador de voluntários dos cuidados domiciliários*. Maputo: Ministério da Saúde, República de Moçambique.

Mondlane, Eduardo. 1969. *The Struggle for Mozambique*. Baltimore, MD: Penguin Books.

Morier-Genoud, Eric. 1996. "Of God and Caesar. The Relation Between Christian Churches & the State in Post-Colonial Mozambique, 1974–81." *Le Fait Missionaire* September (3): 1–79.

Morolake, Odetoyinbo, David Stephens, and Alice Welbourn. 2009. "Greater Involvement of People Living with HIV in Health Care." *Journal of the International AIDS Society* 12 (1): 1–7. https://doi.org/10.1186/1758-2652-12-4.

Moyer, Eileen, and Anita Hardon. 2014. "A Disease Unlike Any Other? Why HIV Remains Exceptional in the Age of Treatment." *Medical Anthropology* 33 (4): 263–69. https://doi.org/10.1080/01459740.2014.890618.

MSF Africa, Department of Public Health at University of Cape Town, and South Africa Provincial Administration of the Western Cape. 2003. *Antiretroviral Therapy in Primary Health Care: Experience of the Khayelitsha Programme in South Africa*. Geneva: World Health Organization.

Muchano, Leonel. 2006. *Tete: Crenças Culturais Ofuscam Esforços de Prevenção e Combate Ao HIV/SIDA Em Changara*. Agencia de Informação de Moçambique, April 26.

Mugyenyi, Peter. 2008. *Genocide by Denial: How Profiteering from HIV/AIDS Killed Millions*. Kampala, Uganda: Fountain.

Mukherjee, Siddhartha. 2000. "Take Your Medicine: Why Cheap AIDS Drugs for Africa Might Be Dangerous." *New Republic*, July 24.

Mulligan, Jessica. 2017. "Biological Citizenship." In *Oxford Bibliography of Anthropology*, edited by John L. Jackson. Oxford University Press. https://oxfordbibliographies.com/view/document/obo-9780199766567/obo-9780199766567-0164.xml.

Mussa, Abdul H., James Pfeiffer, Stephen S. Gloyd, and Kenneth Sherr. 2013. "Vertical Funding, Non-governmental Organizations, and Health System Strengthening: Perspectives of Public Sector Health

Workers in Mozambique." *Human Resources for Health* 11 (1): 26. https://doi.org/10.1186/1478-4491-11-26.

NDPB. 2004. *Poverty and Well-Being in Mozambique: The Second National Assessment*. Maputo: National Directorate of Planning and Budget, Ministry of Planning and Finance, International Food Policy Research Institute, Purdue University.

Neves, Joel Das. 1998a. "A American Board Mission e Os Desafios Do Protestantismo Em Manica e Sofala (Moçambique), ca. 1900–1950." *Lusotopie* 5: 335–43.

———. 1998b. "Economy, Society, and Labour Migration in Central Mozambique, 1930–c. 1965: A Case Study of Manica Province." PhD diss., University of London.

Newell, Sasha. 2006. "Estranged Belongings: A Moral Economy of Theft in Abidjan, Côte d'Ivoire." *Anthropological Theory* 6 (2): 179–203. https://doi.org/10.1177/1463499606065034.

———. 2007. "Pentecostal Witchcraft: Neoliberal Possession and Demonic Discourse in Ivoirian Pentecostal Churches." *Journal of Religion in Africa* 37 (4): 461–90. https://doi.org/10.1163/157006607X230517.

Newitt, M. D. D. 1995. *A History of Mozambique*. Bloomington: Indiana University Press.

Nguyen, Vinh-Kim. 2005. "Antiretroviral Globalism, Biopolitics, and Therapeutic Citizenship." In *Global Assemblages: Technology, Politics, and Ethics as Anthropological Problems*, edited by Aihwa Ong and Stephen Collier, 124–44. Malden: Blackwell Publishing.

———. 2009. "Government-by-Exception: Enrolment and Experimentality in Mass HIV Treatment Programmes in Africa." *Social Theory & Health* 7 (3): 196–217. https://doi.org/10.1057/sth.2009.12.

———. 2010. *The Republic of Therapy: Triage and Sovereignty in West Africa's Time of AIDS*. Durham, NC: Duke University Press.

Nguyen, Vinh-Kim, C. Y. Ako, P. Niamba, A. Sylla, and I. Tiendrebeogo. 2007. "Adherence as Therapeutic Citizenship: Impact of the History of Access to Antiretroviral Drugs on Adherence to Treatment." *AIDS* 21 (Supp. 5): S31–5.

Nguyen, Vinh-Kim, and Karine Peschard. 2003. "Anthropology, Inequality, and Disease: A Review." *Annual Review of Anthropology* 32 (1): 447–74.

Niehaus, Isak. 2007. "Death before Dying: Understanding AIDS Stigma in the South Africa Lowveld." *Journal of Southern African Studies* 33 (4): 816–45.

Nordstrom, Carolyn. 1997. *A Different Kind of War Story*. Philadelphia: University of Pennsylvania Press.

———. 1998. "Terror Warfare and the Medicine of Peace." *Medical Anthropology Quarterly* 12 (1): 103–21.

Notícias. 2006. "Não combate fome com barriga cheia." [No specific date].

O'Laughlin, Bridget. 1996. "From Basic Needs to Safety-Nets: The Rise and Fall of Urban Food-Rationing in Mozambique." *European Journal of Development Research* 8 (1): 200–23. https://doi.org/10.1080/09578819608426658.

O'Laughlin, Bridget. 2000. "Class and the Customary: The Ambiguous Legacy of the Indigenato in Mozambique." *African Affairs* 99 (394): 5–42. https://doi.org/10.1093/afraf/99.394.5.

Obarrio, Juan. 2015. *The Spirit of the Laws in Mozambique*. Chicago: University of Chicago Press. .

Olsen, Bent Steenberg. 2013. "Structures of Stigma: Diagonal AIDS Care and Treatment Abandonment in Mozambique." PhD diss., Roskilde University.

Oomman, Nandini, Michael Bernstein, and Steven Rosenzweig. 2007. *Following the Funding for HIV/AIDS: A Comparative Analysis of the Funding Practices of PEPFAR, the Global Fund and World Bank MAP in Mozambique, Uganda and Zambia*. Washington, DC: Center for Global Development.

———. 2008. *The Numbers Behind the Stories: PEPFAR Funding for Fiscal Years 2004 to 2006*. Washington, DC: Center for Global Development.

Orr, Neil. 2003. *Vida Positiva*. 2nd ed. Maputo: Conselho Nacional de Combate ao HIV/SIDA.

Parish, J. 2000. "From the Body to the Wallet: Conceptualizing Akan Witchcraft at Home and Abroad." *Journal of the Royal Anthropological Institute* 6 (3): 487–500.

Patton, Cindy. 1990. *Inventing AIDS*. New York: Routledge.

Penvenne, Jeanne Marie. 1995. *African Workers and Colonial Racism: Mozambican Strategies and Struggles in Lourenco Marques, 1877–1962*. London: James Currey.

Petryna, Adriana. 2002. *Life Exposed: Biological Citizens after Chernobyl*. Princeton, NJ: Princeton University Press.

Pfeiffer, James. 2002. "African Independent Churches in Mozambique: Healing the Afflictions of Inequality." *Medical Anthropology Quarterly* 16 (2): 176–99.

———. 2003a. "Cash Income, Intrahousehold Cooperative Conflict, and Child Health in Central Mozambique." *Medical Anthropology* 22 (2): 87–130.

———. 2003b. "International NGOs and Primary Health Care in Mozambique: The Need for a New Model of Collaboration." *Social Science and Medicine* 56 (4): 725–38.

———. 2004a. "Condom Social Marketing, Pentecostalism, and Structural Adjustment in Mozambique: A Clash of AIDS Prevention Messages." *Medical Anthropology Quarterly* 18 (1): 77–103.

———. 2004b. "International NGOs in the Mozambique Health Sector: The 'Velvet Glove' of Privatization." In *Unhealthy Health Policy: A Critical Anthropological Examination*, edited by Arachu Castro and Merrill Singer, 43–62. Walnut Creek, CA: AltaMira Press.

———. 2005. "Commodity *Fetichismo*, the Holy Spirit, and the Turn to Pentecostal and African Independent Churches in Central Mozambique." *Culture, Medicine, and Psychiatry* 29 (3): 255–83. https://doi .org/10.1007/s11013-005-9168-3.

———. 2011. "Pentecostalism and AIDS Treatment in Mozambique: Creating New Approaches to HIV Prevention through Anti-Retroviral Therapy." *Global Public Health* 6 (Supp. 2): S163–73. https://doi.org/10 .1080/17441692.2011.605067.

———. 2013. "The Struggle for a Public Sector: PEPFAR in Mozambique." In *When People Come First: Critical Studies in Global Health*, edited by João Biehl and Adriana Petryna, 166–81. Princeton, NJ: Princeton University Press.

———. 2019. "Austerity in Africa Audit Cultures and the Weakening of Public Sector Health Systems." *Focaal* 2019 (83): 51–61. https://doi.org /10.3167/fcl.2019.830105.

Pfeiffer, James, and Rachel Chapman. 2010. "Anthropological Perspectives on Structural Adjustment and Public Health." *Annual Review of Anthropology* 39 (1): 149–65. https://doi.org/10.1146/annurev.anthro .012809.105101.

———. 2019. "NGOs, Austerity, and Universal Health Coverage in Mozambique." *Globalization and Health* 15 (Supp. 1): 1–6. https://doi .org/10.1186/s12992-019-0520-8.

Pfeiffer, James, Sarah Gimbel, Baltazar Chilundo, Stephen Gloyd, Rachel Chapman, and Kenneth Sherr. 2017. "Austerity and the 'Sector-Wide Approach' to Health: The Mozambique Experience." *Social Science & Medicine*, 1–9. https://doi.org/10.1016/j.socscimed.2017.05.008.

Pfeiffer, James, Kenneth Gimbel-Sherr, and Orvalho Joaquim Augusto. 2007. "The Holy Spirit in the Household: Pentecostalism, Gender, and Neoliberalism in Mozambique." *American Anthropologist* 109 (4): 688–700.

Pfeiffer, James, W. Johnson, M. Fort, A. Shakow, A. Hagopian, S. Gloyd, and K. Gimbel-Sherr. 2008. "Strengthening Health Systems in Poor Countries: A Code of Conduct for Nongovernmental Organizations." *American Journal of Public Health* 98 (12): 2134–40.

Phiri, Madalitso Zililo. 2012. "The Political Economy of Mozambique Twenty Years On: A Post-Conflict Success Story?" *South African Journal of International Affairs* 19 (2): 223–45. https://doi.org/10.1080/10220461.2012.707791.

Pickett, Kate, and Richard Wilkinson. 2010. *The Spirit Level: Why Greater Equliaty Makes Societies Stronger.* New York: Bloomsbury Press.

Pierre, Jemima. 2020. "The Racial Vernaculars of Development: A View from West Africa." *American Anthropologist* 122 (1): 86–98. https://doi.org/10.1111/aman.13352.

Pigg, Stacy Leigh. 1996. "The Credible and the Credulous: The Question of 'Villagers Beliefs' in Nepal." *Cultural Anthropology* 11 (2): 160–201.

———. 2001. "Languages of Sex and AIDS in Nepal: Notes of the Social Production of Commensurability." *Cultural Anthropology* 16 (4): 481–541.

Piot, Charles D. 1991. "Of Persons and Things: Some Reflections on African Spheres of Exchange." *Man* 26 (3): 405–24. https://doi.org/10.2307/2803875.

Pitcher, M. Anne. 2002. *Transforming Mozambique: The Politics of Privatization, 1975–2000.* New York: Cambridge University Press.

———. 2006. "Forgetting from Above and Memory from Below: Strategies of Legitimation and Struggle in Postsocialist Mozambique." *Africa* 76 (1): 88–112.

PNCS. 2004. *Guia para o tratamento da infecção pelo HIV no adulto.* Maputo: Programa Nacional de Controle das DTS/SIDA, Direcção Nacional de Saúde, Ministério de Saúde.

Prince, Ruth J. 2007. "Salvation and Tradition—Configurations of Faith in a Time of Death." *Journal of Religion in Africa* 37: 84–115.

———. 2012. "HIV and the Moral Economy of Survival in an East African City." *Medical Anthropology Quarterly* 26 (4): 534–56.

———. 2014a. Introduction to *Making and Unmaking Public Health in Africa: Ethnographic and Historical Perspectives*, 1–51. Athens: Ohio University Press.

———. 2014b. "Precarious Projects: Conversions of (Biomedical) Knowledge in an East African City." *Medical Anthropology* 33 (1): 68–83. https://doi.org/10.1080/01459740.2013.833918.

———. 2015. "Seeking Incorporation? Voluntary Labor and the Ambiguities of Work, Identity, and Social Value in Contemporary Kenya." *African Studies Review* 58 (2): 85–109. https://doi.org/http://dx.doi.org/10.1017/asr.2015.39.

———. 2016. "The Diseased Body and the Global Subject: The Circulation and Consumption of an Iconic AIDS Photograph in East Africa." *Visual Anthropology* 29 (2): 159–86. https://doi.org/10.1080/08949468.2016.1131517.

Prince, Ruth J., Philippe Denis, and Rijk van Dijk. 2009. Introduction to "Engaging Christianities: Negotiating HIV/AIDS, Health, and Social Relations in East and Southern Africa." Special issue, *Africa Today* 56 (1).

Rabinow, Paul. 1992. "Artificiality and Enlightenment: From Sociobiology to Biosociality." In *Incorporations*, edited by Jonathan Crary and Sanford Kwinter, 234–52. New York: Zone Books.

Radcliffe-Brown, Alfred R. 1952. *Structure and Function in Primitive Society: Essays and Addresses*. Glencoe, IL: Free Press.

Ranger, Terence O. 1981. "Godly Medicine: The Ambiguities of Medical Mission in Southeast Tanzania, 1900–1945." *Social Science and Medicine, Part B: Medical Anthropology* 15 (3): 261–77. https://doi.org/10.1016/0160-7987(81)90052-1.

———. 1987. "Religion, Development, and African Christian Identity." In *Religion, Development, and African Identity*, edited by Alan R Petersen, 29–57. Uppsala: Scandinavian Institute of African Studies.

Ransome, Yusuf, Ichiro Kawachi, Sarah Braunstein, and Denis Nash. 2016. "Structural Inequalities Drive Late HIV Diagnosis: The Role of Black Racial Concentration, Income Inequality, Socioeconomic Deprivation, and HIV Testing." *Health and Place* 42: 148–58. https://doi.org/10.1016/j.healthplace.2016.09.004.

Redfield, Peter. 2008. "Doctors Without Borders and the Moral Economy of Pharmaceuticals." In *Human Rights in Crisis*, edited by Alice Bullard, 129–44. Hampshire, UK: Ashgate.

———. 2013. *Life in Crisis: The Ethical Journey of Doctors Without Borders*. Berkeley: University of California Press.

Reed, Joel Christian. 2014. "The Disintegration of the Day Hospitals." In *Medical Anthropology in Global Africa*, edited by Kathryn Rhine, John M. Janzen, Glenn Adams, and Heather Aldersey, 63–70. Lawrence: University of Kansas.

———. 2018. *Landscapes of Activism: Civil Society, HIV and AIDS Care in Northern Mozambique*. New Brunswick, NJ: Rutgers University Press.

Rees, Tobias. 2014. "Humanity/Plan; or, on the 'Stateless' Today (Also Being an Anthropology of Global Health)." *Cultural Anthropology* 29 (3): 457–78. https://doi.org/10.14506/ca29.3.02.

Reis, Bruno C., and Pedro A. Oliveira. 2012. "Cutting Heads or Winning Hearts: Late Colonial Portuguese Counterinsurgency and the Wiriyamu Massacre of 1972." *Civil Wars* 14 (1): 80–103. https://doi.org/10.1080/13698249.2012.654690.

Richardson, Eugene T. 2019. "On the Coloniality of Global Public Health." *Medicine Anthropology Theory* 6 (4): 101–18. https://doi.org/10.17157/mat.6.4.761.

Richey, Lisa Ann. 2011. "Antiviral but Postnatal? ARVs and Reproductive Health: The View from a South African Township." In *Reproduction, Globalization, and the State: New Theoretical and Ethnographic Perspectives*, edited by Carole H. Browner and Carolyn Fishel Sargent, 68–82. Durham, NC: Duke University Press.

Richey, Lisa Ann, and Stefano Ponte. 2011. *Brand Aid: Shopping Well to Save the World*. Minneapolis: University of Minnesota Press. https://doi.org/10.1017/asr.2013.63.

Rödlach, A. 2009. "Home-Based Care for People Living with AIDS in Zimbabwe: Voluntary Caregivers' Motivations and Concerns." *African Journal of AIDS Research (AJAR)* 8: 423–31. https://doi.org/10.2989/AJAR.2009.8.4.6.1043.

Roesch, Otto. 1992. "Renamo and the Peasantry in Southern Mozambique: A View from Gaza Province." *Canadian Journal of African Studies* 26 (3): 462–84.

Rose, Nikolas. 1996. "The Death of the Social? Re-Figuring the Territory of Government." *Economy and Society* 25 (3): 327–56. https://doi.org/10.1080/03085149600000018.

Ross, Edward Alsworth. 1925. *Report on Employment of Native Labor in Portuguese Africa*. New York: Abbott Press.

Ruckert, Arne, and Ronald Labonté. 2017. "Health Inequities in the Age of Austerity: The Need for Social Protection Policies." *Social Science and Medicine* 187: 306–11. https://doi.org/10.1016/j.socscimed.2017.03.029.

Sangaramoorthy, Thurka. 2014. *Treating AIDS: Politics of Difference, Paradox of Prevention.* New Brunswick, NJ: Rutgers University Press.

———. 2018. "Chronicity, Crisis, and the 'End of AIDS.'" *Global Public Health* 13 (8): 982–96. https://doi.org/10.1080/17441692.2018.1423701.

Santos, Fr. João dos. 1999. *Etiópia oriental e vária história de cousas cotáveis do Oriente.* Lisbon: Comissão Nacional Para as Comemorações dos Descobrimentos Portugueses.

Sardan, J. P. Olivier De. 1999. "A Moral Economy of Corruption in Africa?" *Journal of Modern African Studies* 37 (1): 25–52.

Schafer, Jessica. 1998. "'A Baby Who Does Not Cry Will Not Be Suckled': AMODEG and the Reintegration of Demobilised Soldiers." *Journal of Southern African Studies* 24 (1): 207–22.

Scheper-Hughes, Nancy. 1992. *Death without Weeping: The Violence of Everyday Life in Brazil.* Berkeley: University of California Press.

———. 1993. "Hungry Bodies, Medicine, and the State: Toward a Critical Psychological Anthropology." In *New Directions in Psychological Anthropology,* 221–48. Cambridge, UK: Cambridge University Press. https://doi.org/10.1017/CBO9780511621857.012.

Scheper-Hughes, Nancy, and Margaret M. Lock. 1987. "The Mindful Body: A Prolegomenon to Future Work in Medical Anthropology." *Medical Anthropology Quarterly* 1 (1): 6–41.

Scherz, C. S. 2014. *Having People, Having Heart: Charity, Sustainable Development, and Problems of Dependence in Central Uganda.* Chicago: University of Chicago Press.

Scott, James C. 1976. *The Moral Economy of the Peasant: Rebellion and Subsistence in Southeast Asia.* New Haven, CT: Yale University Press.

Scott, James C. 1998. *Seeing Like a State: How Certain Schemes to Improve the Human Condition Have Failed.* Yale Agrarian Studies. New Haven, CT: Yale University Press.

Seeley, Janet, Charlotte H. Watts, Susan Kippax, Steven Russell, Lori Heise, and Alan Whiteside. 2012. "Addressing the Structural Drivers of HIV: A Luxury or Necessity for Programmes?" *Journal of the International AIDS Society* 15 (Supp. 1): 15–18. https://doi.org/10.7448/IAS.15.3.17397.

Seibert, Gerhard. 2005. "'But the Manifestation of the Spirit Is Given to Every Man to Profit Withal': Zion Churches in Mozambique since the Early 20th Century." *Le Fait Missionaire* 17: 103–28.

Seidel, Gill. 1993. "The Competing Discourses of HIV/AIDS in Sub-Saharan Africa: Discourses of Rights and Empowerment vs. Discourses of Control and Exclusion." *Social Science & Medicine* 36 (3): 175–94.

Serwadda, D., R. D. Mugerwa, N. K. Sewankambo, A. Lwegaba, J. W. Carswell, G. B. Kirya, A. C. Bayley, R. G. Downing, R. S. Tedder, and S. A. Clayden. 1985. "Slim Disease: A New Disease in Uganda and Its Association with HTLV-III Infection." *Lancet* 2 (8460): 849–52.

Setel, Philip. 1999. *A Plague of Paradoxes: AIDS, Culture, and Demography in Northern Tanzania*. Chicago: University of Chicago Press.

SETSAN. 2008. "Malnutrição Crónica Agrava-Se No País." www.setsan.org.mz/Index.htm.

Shamasunder, Sriram, Seth M. Holmes, Tinashe Goronga, Hector Carrasco, Elyse Katz, Raphael Frankfurter, and Salmaan Keshavjee. 2020. "COVID-19 Reveals Weak Health Systems by Design: Why We Must Re-make Global Health in This Historic Moment." *Global Public Health* 15(7): 1083–89. https://doi.org/10.1080/17441692.2020.1760915.

Shapiro, Martin. 1983. "Medicine in the Service of Colonialism: Medical Care in Portuguese Africa, 1885–1974." PhD diss., University of California, Los Angeles.

Sherr, Kenneth, Antonio Mussa, Baltazar Chilundo, Sarah Gimbel, James Pfeiffer, Amy Hagopian, and Stephen Gloyd. 2012. "Brain Drain and Health Workforce Distortions in Mozambique." *PLoS ONE* 7 (4). https://doi.org/10.1371/journal.pone.0035840.

Shevitz, Abby H. 1999. "Elevated Resting Energy Expenditure among HIV-Seropositive Persons Receiving Highly Active Antiretroviral Therapy." *AIDS* 13 (11): 1351–57. https://doi.org/10.1097/00002030-199907300-00012.

Shore, Cris, and Susan Wright, eds. 1997. *Anthropology of Policy: Critical Perspectives on Governance and Power*. New York: Routledge.

Shweder, Richard, and Edmund Bourne. 1982. "Does the Concept of the Person Vary Cross-Culturally?" In *Cultural Conceptions of Mental Health and Therapy*, edited by Anthony J. Marsella and Geoffrey M. White, 97–137. Dordrecht: Reidel.

Siegel, Brian. 2013. "Neo-Pentecostalism in Black Africa." Anthropology Presentations, Paper 1. http://scholarexchange.furman.edu/ant-presentatons/1.

Simone, A. M. 2004. "People as Infrastructure: Intersecting Fragments in Johannesburg." *Public Culture* 16 (3): 407–29.

Smith, Daniel Jordan. 2003. "Patronage, Per Diems and the 'Workshop Mentality': The Practice of Family Planning Programs in Southeastern Nigeria." *World Development* 31 (4): 703–15. https://doi.org/10.1016 /S0305-750X(03)00006-8.

———. 2014. *AIDS Doesn't Show Its Face: Inequality, Morality, and Social Change in Nigeria.* Chicago: University of Chicago Press.

Sontag, Deborah, Sharon LaFraniere, and Michael Wines. 2004. "Early Tests for US in Its Global Fight on AIDS." *New York Times,* July 14.

Sparke, Matthew. 2014. "Health." In *The SAGE Handbook of Human Geography,* edited by Roger Lee, Noel Castree, Rob Kitchin, Vicky Lawson, Anssi Paasi, Chris Philo, Sarah Radcliffe, Susan M. Roberts, and Charles Withers, 680–704. Los Angeles: SAGE.

———. 2017. "Austerity and the Embodiment of Neoliberalism as Ill-Health: Towards a Theory of Biological Sub-Citizenship." *Social Science & Medicine* 187 (August): 287–95. https://doi.org/10.1016/j.socscimed .2016.12.027.

———. 2020. "Neoliberal Regime Change and the Remaking of Global Health: From Rollback Disinvestment to Rollout Reinvestment and Reterritorialization." *Review of International Political Economy* 27 (1): 48–74. https://doi.org/10.1080/09692290.2019.1624382.

Stevens, W., S. Kaye, and T. Corrah. 2004. "Antiretroviral Therapy in Africa." *British Medical Journal* 328 (January 31): 280–82.

Stillwaggon, Eileen. 2002. "HIV/AIDS in Africa: Fertile Terrain." *Journal of Development Studies* 38 (6): 1–22.

———. 2006. "The Ecology of Poverty: Nutrition, Parasites, and Vulnerability to HIV/AIDS." In *AIDS, Poverty, and Hunger: Challenges and Responses,* edited by Stuart Gillespie, 167–80. Washington, DC: International Food Policy Research Institute.

Stonington, Scott D., Seth M. Holmes, Helena Hansen, Jeremy A. Greene, Keith A. Wailoo, Debra Malina, Stephen Morrissey, Paul E. Farmer, and Michael G. Marmot. 2018. "Case Studies in Social Medicine—Attending to Structural Forces in Clinical Practice." *New England Journal of Medicine.* 379 (20): 1958–61. https://doi.org/10.1056/NEJMms1814262.

Strathern, Marilyn. 2000. *Audit Cultures: Anthropological Studies into Accountablity, Ethics, and the Academy.* London: Routledge.

Sullivan, Noelle. 2011. "Mediating Abundance and Scarcity: Implementing an HIV/AIDS-Targeted Project within a Government Hospital in

Tanzania." *Medical Anthropology* 30: 202–21. https://doi.org/10.1080 /01459740.2011.552453.

Swartz, Alison. 2013. "Legacy, Legitimacy, and Possibility: An Exploration of Community Health Worker Experience across the Generations in Khayelitsha, South Africa." *Medical Anthropology Quarterly* 27: 139–54. https://doi.org/10.1111/maq.12020.

Swidler, A, and S C Watkins. 2009. "'Teach a Man to Fish': The Doctrine of Sustainability and Its Effects on Three Strata of Malawian Society." *World Development* 37 (7): 1182–96. https://doi.org/10.1016/j.worlddev .2008.11.002.

Taussig, Michael T. 1980a. "Reification and the Consciousness of the Patient." *Social Science & Medicine* 14B: 3–13.

———. 1980b. *The Devil and Commodity Fetishism in Latin America.* Chapel Hill: University of North Carolina Press.

———. 1986. *Shamanism, Colonialism, and the Wild Man: A Study in Terror and Healing.* Chicago: University of Chicago Press.

Taylor, Rex, and Annelie Rieger. 1984. "Rudolf Virchow on the Typhus Epidemic in Upper Silesia : An Introduction and Translation." *Sociology of Health and Illness* 6 (2): 201–18.

Thompson, E. P. 1971. "The Moral Economy of the English Crowd in the Eighteenth Century." *Past and Present* 50 (February): 76–136.

Ticktin, Miriam. 2011. *Casualties of Care: Immigration and the Politics of Humanitarianism in France.* Berkeley: University of California Press.

Treichler, Paula A. 1999. *How to Have Theory in an Epidemic: Cultural Chronicles of AIDS.* Durham, NC: Duke University Press.

Umberg, Jennifer. 2015. "The Journey of a Voucher in Mozambique." World Food Program.

UNAIDS. 2002. *Report on the Global HIV/AIDS Epidemic.* Geneva: UNAIDS.

———. 2010. *Global Report: UNAIDS Report on the Global AIDS Epidemic.* Geneva: UNAIDS.

———. 2013. *Global Update on HIV Treatment 2013: Results, Impacts, and Opportunities.* Geneva: UNAIDS.

———. 2020. *Seizing the Moment: Tackling Entrenched Inequalities to End Epidemics.* Geneva: UNAIDS.

United Nations. 1996. *Report of the World Summit for Social Development.* New York: United Nations.

Vansina, Jan. 1990. *Paths in the Rainforests: Toward a History of Political Tradition in Equatorial Africa*. Madison: University of Wisconsin Press.

Vaughan, Megan. 1991. *Curing Their Ills: Colonial Power and African Illness*. Stanford, CA: Stanford University Press.

Villarosa, Linda. 2017. "America's Hidden HIV Epidemic: Why Do America's Black Gay and Bisexual Men Have a Higher HIV Rate Than Any Country in the World?" *New York Times*, June 6.

Vines, Alex, and Ken Wilson. 1995. "Churches and the Peace Process in Mozambique." In *The Christian Churches and the Democratisation of Africa*, edited by Paul Gifford, 130–48. Leiden: Brill.

Waal, Alex De, and A. Whiteside. 2003. "New Variant Famine: AIDS and Food Crisis in Southern Africa." *Lancet* 362 (9391): 1234–37.

Waite, Gloria. 1992. "Public Health in Pre-Colonial East Africa." In *The Social Basis of Health and Healing in Africa*, edited by Steven Feierman and John M Janzen, 212–33. Berkeley: University of California Press.

Waitzkin, Howard. 2006. "One and a Half Centuries of Forgetting and Rediscovering : Virchow's Lasting Contributions to Social Medicine." *Social Medicine* 1 (1): 5–10.

Weiser, S. D., S. L. Young, C. R. Cohen, M. B. Kushel, A. C. Tsai, P. C. Tien, A. M. Hatcher, E. A. Frongillo, and D. R. Bangsberg. 2011. "Conceptual Framework for Understanding the Bidirectional Links between Food Insecurity and HIV/AIDS." *American Journal of Clinical Nutrition* 94 (6): 1729S–39S. https://doi.org/10.3945/ajcn.111.012070.

Weiser, Sheri, Elizabeth A. Bukusi, Rachel L. Steinfeld, Edward A. Frongillo, Elly Weke, Shari L. Dworkin, Kyle Pusateri, et al. 2015. "Shamba Maisha: Randomized Controlled Trial of an Agricultural and Finance Intervention to Improve HIV Health Outcomes in Kenya." *AIDS* 29 (14): 1889–94. https://doi:10.1097/QAD.0000000 000000781.

Wendland, Claire L. 2010. *A Heart for the Work: Journeys through an African Medical School*. Chicago: University of Chicago Press.

———. 2012. "Moral Maps and Medical Imaginaries: Clinical Tourism at Malawi's College of Medicine." *American Anthropologist* 114 (1): 108–22. https://doi.org/10.1111/j.1548-1433.2011.01400.x.

Werner, David, Carol Thuman, and Jane Maxwell. 2017. *Where There Is No Doctor*. Berkeley: Hesperian Health Guides.

West, Harry G. 2001. "Sorcery of Construction and Socialist Moderniza-
    tion: Ways of Understanding Postcolonial Mozambique." *American
    Ethnologist* 28 (1): 119–50.
———. 2005. *Kupilikula: Governance and the Invisible Realm in Mozam-
    bique*. Chicago: University of Chicago Press.
White, Sarah. 2002. "Thinking Race, Thinking Development." *Third
    World Quarterly* 23 (3): 407–19.
Whyte, Susan Reynolds. 1997. *Questioning Misfortune: The Pragmatics
    of Uncertainty in Eastern Uganda*. New York: Cambridge University
    Press.
———. 2002. "Subjectivity and Subjunctivity: Hoping for Health in
    Eastern Uganda." In *Postcolonial Subjectivities in Africa*, edited by
    Richard P. Werbner, 171–90. London: Zed Books.
———. 2014. *Second Chances: Surviving AIDS in Uganda*. Durham, NC:
    Duke University Press.
Whyte, Susan Reynolds, M. A. Whyte, L. Meinert, and J. Twebaze. 2013.
    "Therapeutic Clientship: Belonging in Uganda's Projectified Landscape
    of AIDS Care." In *When People Come First: Critical Studies in Global
    Health*, edited by João Biehl and Adriana Petryna, 140–65. Princeton,
    NJ: Princeton University Press.
Williams, David, and Chiquita Collins. 2004. "Reparations: A Viable
    Strategy to Address the Enigma of African American Health."
    American Behavioral Scientist 47 (7): 977–1000. https://doi.org/10
    .1177/0002764203261074.
Williams, Rosa Janet. 2013. "Creating a Healthy Colonial State in
    Mozambique, 1885–1915." PhD diss., University of Chicago.
Wilson, Phill, Kai Wright, and Michael T. Isbell. 2008. "Left Behind:
    Black America; A Neglected Priority in the Global AIDS Epidemic."
    Los Angeles: Black AIDS Institute.
World Bank. 1989. *Mozambique: Public Expenditure Review*. Washington
    D.C: World Bank.
———. 2007."*Beating the Odds: Sustaining Inclusion in a Growing
    Economy*. Washington, DC: World Bank Africa Region Poverty
    Reduction and Economic Management.
World Health Organization. 2020. "WHO: Access to HIV Medicines
    Severely Impacted by COVID-19 as AIDS Response Stalls." www.who
    .int/news-room/detail/06-07-2020-who-access-to-hiv-medicines
    -severely-impacted-by-covid-19-as-aids-response-stalls.

Yager, Jessica E., Suneetha Kadiyala, and Sheri D. Weiser. 2011. "HIV/AIDS, Food Supplementation and Livelihood Programs in Uganda: A Way Forward?" *PLoS ONE* 6 (10): 18–22. https://doi.org/10.1371/journal.pone.0026117.

Zwi, A. B., and A. J. R. Cabral. 1991. "Identifying 'High Risk Situations' for Preventing AIDS." *British Medical Journal* 303 (6816): 1527–29. https://doi.org/10.1136/bmj.303.6816.1527.

Index

Adélia, 161–62, 165, 170–71, 173

Africa: "declarations of dependence" of people in Africa, 187–88; the disparagement of African "backwardness," 112; famine in southern Africa ("new variant famine"), 180–81; healing in southeastern Africa, 188; idioms of hunger in, 11; inability of African governments to control macroeconomic processes, 75–76; northern intervention in, 193; obstacles to HIV/AIDS treatment in, 174; and personhood, 6–7; racist and classist assumptions concerning Africans and AIDS treatment programs, 166; redistributive policies in southern Africa, 236–37n55. *See also* sub-Saharan Africa

African Independent Churches (AICs), 41, 41*fig.*, 43, 44, 124

African Network of AIDS Service Organizations, 82

AIDS activists/activism, 63, 198–99

AIDS economy, the, 5–6, 45, 51, 78, 80, 114–15, 122, 151; the "business of AIDS," 192–93; characteristics of, 177; conspiracy theories and suspicions in, 73–74; cosmopolitan modernity of, 101; fieldwork concerning, 23–25, 220n76; positive living (*Vida Positiva*) in the AIDS economy, 15–17

"AIDS kills" (*SIDA Mata*): fatalism of, 63; fear-based messages of, 62; and the stakes of visibility, 58–62, 67–68

AIDS Support Organization, The (TASO), 82, 228n1

AIDS testimonials, 96–97, 157; Batista's testimonial, 102–3; Bruno's testimonial, 98–99, 100*fig.*; and the experience of rebirth, 99–100; Fernando's testimonial, 97–98; and living positively, 101

alcohol/drinking, 72, 90, 162

"all I eat is ARVs" comment, 11–12, 79, 177

Alma Ata Declaration (1978), 144

antibiotics, 139, 153–54, 160

antiretroviral medications (ARVs), 2, 4, 9, 10, 99, 110, 115, 142, 150, 152, 160, 165, 194; access to, 168, 174–75;

192; as the largest funder of AIDS treatment, 149–50
Prince, Ruth, 218–19n64
privatization, 75
Product Red, 216n5
profetes (prophet-healers), 8, 9, 42*fig.*, 52, 54, 80–81, 95, 227n12, 229n14; as pagan, 124. *See also* Lucia (a *profete*)
prostitution, 59–60
Protestants, 54; Protestant missions, 40–41

race, and colonialism, 14
racism, 199
Rees, Tobias, 198
Republic of Therapy, The: Triage and Sovereignty in West Africa's Time of AIDS (Nguyen), 75
Rhodesia, 39; Southern Rhodesia, 38–39, 41
Rita, 50–51, 52, 55, 58–59, 76–77, 78, 80, 81, 115–16, 183, 194
Ross, Edward, 32

SARS-CoV-2, 203
Scheper-Hughes, Nancy, 176
Scherz, China, 7, 187
"scientific socialism," 38
Scott, James, 79, 218n63
"Scramble for Africa," the, 31, 40
Severino, 126
sex/reproduction/fertility, 164; condom use and disclosure of HIV status, 109; and infertility, 108, 227n23; mixed messages concerning, 107–9; preaching of safe sex among associations yet toleration of pregnancies, 108; unprotected sex, 164
smoking/tobacco use, 72, 90, 162
socialism, 47; scientific, 46
social relationships, 128–29, 194
Sofala province, 33
solidarity, 103, 193
South Africa, 38–39, 41, 60; Basic Income Grant of, 202
sovereignty, 76
spirits: ancestral (*vadzimu*), 8, 130, 168; evil (*espírito mau*), 8
spiritual healing, and biomedicine, 94–95

subjectivity: cosmopolitan, 95; definition of, 218n55; "technologies" of, 174
sub-Saharan Africa, 235n39; healing in as "public," 8; intersection of the AIDS epidemic with a lack of infrastructure in, 144; privatization program in, 6
subsistence, as a moral claim, 76–81
Suraia, 108–9, 115
Suzana, 24–25, 103, 167

Takashinga (We Were Brave), 82–83, 88, 91, 93, 97, 134; reasons for the acrimonious split within, 105–6
Tanzania, families caring for loved ones suffering from AIDS in, 226n6
TARV, 215–16n4
Taussig, Michael, 7
"technologies of subjectivity," 174
técnicos de medicina, 150
Teresa, 55–58, 194–95
testemunha concept, 156–57, 160
TextÁfrica, 18, 18*fig.*, 21–22, 35, 105, 219–20n73
TexLom, 35
Tex Moque, 35
"therapeutic congregations," 27, 122
"therapy managing groups," 224n11
Thompson, E. P., 15–16
Tomas, 61, 112–13
tratamento observado direitamente (TOD), 157, 160
tuberculosis, 133

United Nations, 44, 222n60
United States, 7, 165, 225n31; social welfare reform in (1980s), 173–74
Upper Silesia, typhus epidemic in, 199
uroi (sorcery/an evil spirit [*espírito mau*]), 8, 55, 56, 87, 101, 130
USAID, 139, 173, 183

"vertical" versus "horizontal" programming, 149–50, 230n8
Vida Positiva (positive living), 15, 16, 51, 62–64, 65*fig.*, 66–67, 95, 102, 113, 115, 165, 195, 227n12; assumption in that AIDS patients could no longer reproduce, 164; booklet of, 155–56; doctrine of, 103; facts of, 161–65;

CALIFORNIA SERIES IN PUBLIC ANTHROPOLOGY

Founded in 1893,
UNIVERSITY OF CALIFORNIA PRESS
publishes bold, progressive books and journals
on topics in the arts, humanities, social sciences,
and natural sciences—with a focus on social
justice issues—that inspire thought and action
among readers worldwide.

The UC PRESS FOUNDATION
raises funds to uphold the press's vital role
as an independent, nonprofit publisher, and
receives philanthropic support from a wide
range of individuals and institutions—and from
committed readers like you. To learn more, visit
ucpress.edu/supportus.